NEUROSCIENCE INTELLIGENCE UNIT

NEUROBIOLOGICAL MECHANISMS OF OPIATE WITHDRAWAL

Rafael Maldonado, M.D., Ph.D.
Pharmacochimie Moléculaire et Structurale
Paris, France

Luis Stinus, Ph.D.
Université de Bordeaux II
Bordeaux Cédex, France

George F. Koob, Ph.D.
The Scripps Research Institute
La Jolla, California, U.S.A.

CHAPMAN & HALL
IⓉP An International Thomson Publishing Company

New York • Albany • Bonn • Boston • Cincinnati • Detroit • London • Madrid • Melbourne •
Mexico City • Pacific Grove • Paris • San Francisco • Singapore • Tokyo • Toronto • Washington

R.G. LANDES COMPANY
AUSTIN

NEUROSCIENCE INTELLIGENCE UNIT

NEUROBIOLOGICAL MECHANISMS OF OPIATE WITHDRAWAL

R.G. LANDES COMPANY
Austin, Texas, U.S.A.

U.S. and Canada Copyright © 1996 R.G. Landes Company and Chapman & Hall

Please address all inquiries to the Publishers:
R.G. Landes Company, 909 Pine Street, Georgetown, Texas, U.S.A. 78626
Phone: 512/ 863 7762; FAX: 512/ 863 0081

North American distributor:
Chapman & Hall, 115 Fifth Avenue, New York, New York, U.S.A. 10003

U.S. and Canada ISBN: 0-412-11061-X

Library of Congress Cataloging-in-Publication Data

Maldonado, Rafael, 1961-
    Neurobiological mechanisms of opiate withdrawal / Rafael Maldonado, Luis Stinus, George F. Koob.
        p. cm. — (Neuroscience intelligence unit)
    Includes bibliographical references and index.
    ISBN 1-57059-347-7 (alk. paper), ISBN 0-412-11061-X (alk. paper)
    1. Drug withdrawal symptoms. 2. Opioids--Pathophysiology. 3. Narcotic habit--Pathophysiology. 4. Neurotoxicology.   I. Sinus, Luis. II. Koob, George F. III. Title. IV. Series.
        [DNLM: 1. Substance Withdrawal Syndrom--physiopathology. 2. Narcotics--adverse effects. 3. Nervous System--drug effects. WM284 M244n 1996]
RC568.045M45 1996   616.86'32--dc20
DNLM/DLC   96-8139
for Library of Congress   CIP

Publisher's Note

R.G. Landes Company publishes six book series: *Medical Intelligence Unit, Molecular Biology Intelligence Unit, Neuroscience Intelligence Unit, Tissue Engineering Intelligence Unit, Biotechnology Intelligence Unit* and *Environmental Intelligence Unit.* The authors of our books are acknowledged leaders in their fields and the topics are unique. Almost without exception, no other similar books exist on these topics.

Our goal is to publish books in important and rapidly changing areas of medicine for sophisticated researchers and clinicians. To achieve this goal, we have accelerated our publishing program to conform to the fast pace in which information grows in biomedical science. Most of our books are published within 90 to 120 days of receipt of the manuscript. We would like to thank our readers for their continuing interest and welcome any comments or suggestions they may have for future books.

Deborah Muir Molsberry
Publications Director
R.G. Landes Company

CONTENTS

AUTHOR BIOGRAPHIES

DR. RAFAEL MALDONADO

Dr. Rafael Moldonado earned his M.D and Ph.D in Neuropsychopharmacology at the School of Medicine of the University of Cadiz (Spain) working on the effects of benzodiazepines and anti-depressants on morphine dependence directed by Professor J. Gibert-Rahola. He earned his Ph.D in Molecular Pharmacochemistry at the School of Pharmacy of the University René Descartes (Paris, France) working on the participation of the endogenous opioid system on the development of opiate dependence directed by Professor B.P. Roques and Professor J. Feger. As a postdoctorate fellow at The Scripps Research Institute (La Jolla, California), directed by Professor G.F. Koob, his interests in drug dependence were cultivated, which led to the study of cocaine self-administration and the neuroanatomical substrate of opioid dependence. After one and a half years in the USA, Dr. Maldonado moved to the laboratory of Molecular Pharmacochemistry of INSERM (U 266) where he obtained a permanent position as scientific researcher (Chargé de Recherches, CR-1). He is currently studying the interactions between the opioid and cholecystokinergic systems in the development of opiate dependence and affective disorders. He is project leader of two cooperative programs of the Commission of the European Communities aimed at the study of opiate dependence and affective disorders: the Biomedical and Health Research Programme and the PECO Programme for Cooperation in Science and Technology with Central and Eastern European Countries and with New Independent States of the Former Soviet Union. He has been a visiting researcher in the Addiction Research Center (Baltimore, USA), the Department of Biochemistry of the Medical School of the University of Montreal (Canada) and the German Cancer Research Center (Heidelberg, Germany). He won the Almirall Award and the Upjohn Award for excellence in research from the Spanish Society of Pharmacology.

DR. LUIS STINUS

Dr. Luis Stinus earned his Ph.D at the University of Bordeaux I (Laboratory of Psychophysiology, Professor B. Cardo) working on the involvement of monoaminergic neuronal systems in intracranial self-stimulation. He entered the Centre National de la Recherche Scientifique (France) in 1970 as a permanent scientific researcher. He was a predoctoral fellow in the laboratory of Neuropharmacology at the Collège de France (Paris) directed by Professor J. Glowinski in 1971-72, and a postdoctoral fellow at the University of Cambridge (England) in the Department of Psychology directed by Professor S. Iversen in 1979, at Harvard Medical School in the Department of Neuroanatomy (Cambridge, USA) under the direction of Professor W. Nauta in 1980-81 and at The Scripps Research Institute (La Jolla, California), Department of Neuropharmacology, under the direction of Professor G.F. Koob during several periods from 1985 to 1992. He discovered (with Drs. A.M. Theirry and J. Glowinski) the dopaminergic innervation of the frontal cortex; he studied the substance P, neurotensin, opioid and GABA regulation of mesolimbic dopaminergic neurons; and in the last 8 years his main interest was focused on the neurophysiological mechanisms involved in behavioral sensitization, tolerance and dependence induced by repeated application of psychostimulant and opiate drugs. At present he is the Director of the Laboratory of "Neuropsychobiologie des desadaptations" of the Medical School of the University of Bordeaux II (France).

Professor G.F. Koob

Dr. George F. Koob is Director of the Division of Psychopharmacology and a Member (Professor) in the Department of Neuropharmacology at The Scripps Research Institute and Adjunct Professor of Psycology and Psychiatry at the University of California, San Diego. Dr. Koob received his Bachelor of Science degree from Pennsylvania State University and his Ph.D in Behavioral Physiology from the Johns Hopkins University. He began his postdoctoral studies in neurophysiology, neurochemistry, and psychopharmacology at the Walter Reed Army Institute of Research, and he continued his postdoctoral fellowship with Dr. Susan D. Iversen at the Department of Experimental Psychology and Dr. Leslie Iversen at the Medical Research Council Neurochemical Pharmacology Unit of the University of Cambridge. He has maintained an active collaboration since 1977 with Dr. Michael Le Moal, Dr. Luis Stinus, Dr. Hervé Simon and Dr. Martine Cador at the Université de Bordeaux II. An authority on addiction and stress, Dr. Koob has published over 300 scientific papers and has received funding for his research from The National Institutes of Health, including The National Institute on Drug Addiction (NIDA) and The National Institute on Alcohol Abuse and Alcoholism (NIAAA) where he is a Merit Awardee. His current research is focused on the exploration of the neurobiological basis for the neuroadaptation associated with drug dependence and stress. He is the United States editor of *Pharmacology Biochemistry and Behavior,* and he is the Director of the NIAAA Alcohol Center at The Scripps Research Institute. There, he has trained over 30 postdoctoral and 7 predoctoral fellows in his neuropharmacology laboratory. He has won four excellence in teaching awards at the University of California, San Diego, and he won the Daniel Efron Award for excellence in research from the American College of Neuropsychopharmacology.

PREFACE

The first section of this book describes some general aspects of opiate dependence. The first chapter includes a brief historical and modern description, and the second one explains the different models currently used to investigate the physical and motivational components of opiate dependence. The neurobiological aspects of opiate withdrawal are described in a second section. First, several important neurophysiological adaptive processes occurring during opiate dependence, such as changes on adenylyl cyclase pathway, c-fos expression or glucose utilization, are reported. Another chapter addresses the processes of homologous and heterologous regulation occurring on different neurotransmitter systems that have been found using classical and modern neurochemistry techniques. The participation of different brain structures in the expression of opiate withdrawal and the involvement of several endogenous peptides acting as antiopiates are also described in this section. The last part of this book addresses several basic aspects more directly related to the clinical perspectives of opiate dependence. The relationships between sensitization, tolerance and withdrawal, which are crucial to the maintenance of opiate addiction, are discussed. A chapter is dedicated to the description of the classical compounds currently used as well as the new expectations to the treatment of opiate withdrawal. Two possible future new treatments are presented: the use of enkephalin catabolism inhibitors and transcutaneous electrical stimulation. The last chapter explains a theory postulated from basic research studies, the opponent process theory of motivation, that has important implications in the research of a rational therapeutic approach to the treatment of opiate addiction.

Acknowledgments

We would like to thank the Molecular and Experimental Medicine word processing unit (Julie Koehler, Supervisor) for their help in manuscript preparation, Mike Arends for help in library research, Pat Brennan for administrative assistance, Professor Bernard Roques for help with the section on inhibitors of enkephalin metabolism, and Dr. Gery Schulteis and Dr. Serge Ahmed for their help on the sensitization chapter. This work was supported in part by NIH grant DA 04043 to G.F. Koob, and grants from the Biomed and Health Research Programme of the European Commission #PL931721 and Ministere de la Recherche et de la Technologie, Toxicomanies 94.V.0264 to Professor Bernard Roques.

CHAPTER 1

HISTORICAL ASPECTS

Opiates are drugs derived from extracts of the juice of the opium poppy and have been used medically for thousands of years. References to the use of poppy extracts with opiate-like actions have been found in the Bible.[1] One of the first references to the medical use of opium was by the Greek Theophrastus who, at the beginning of the third century B.C., spoke of mekoneion.[1] Parcelus (1490-1540), a famous physician of the middle ages, used opium boldly, and his followers were equally enthusiastic.[1] Thomas Sydenham, one of the great physicians of the 17th century, wrote in describing a series of dysentery epidemics in 1669-1672: "And here I cannot but break out in praise of the great God, the giver of all good things, who hath granted to the human race, as a comfort in their affliction, no medicine of the value of opium, either in regard to the number of diseases it can control, or its efficiency in extirpating them."[2]

However, equally early along with the description of opiate medical actions, withdrawal from opiates was described. One of the earliest descriptions of opiate withdrawal was described in 1700 by a Dr. John Jones who detailed the withdrawal associated with cessation of chronic use of opium. In chapter 23 of *The Mysteries of Opium Revealed*,[3] he writes,

The Explication of the Effects of Leaving Off Opium, After a Long and Lavish Use Thereof

I. Great, and even intolerable Distresses, Anxieties, and Depressions of Spirits, do happen: (1) Because the sensitive Soul, who is so much comforted, diverted; and supported by the habitual and dearly beloved pleasure that opium causes, being suddenly deprived thereof, (by which it was mainly sustain'd) is exceedingly disappointed and cast down. (2) Because he now labours under the sore burthen of the three contractions, so that every thing seems, and is really more grievous to him for now it acts as one in pain or grief, and every thing affects him more smartly proportionable to the compression caused thereby of the animal spirits, unless he returns to the pleasure of opium, which elevates it again; or uses generous wine, as its substitute, tho' it does not equal it, either in the intenseness or duration of the pleasure, unless repeated (as I have some where directed) once in half an hours, or an hours, in a moderate manner, which causes a continuance of the pleasure, tho' it cannot equal the intenseness of that of opium, which therefore has the greater effects.

II. A return of all diseases, pains and disasters, must happen generally, because the opium takes them off by a bare diversion of the sense thereof by pleasure.

III. Dangerous loosenesses happen sometimes, because the sensation grows more grievous; for, as the pleasant sensation caused by opium, takes away the perception of the irritation of humours, so the grievance of losing and pleasure causing contraction, makes all sensation smarter, and consequently more irritating, so that the humours have thereby more of the effect of purgers, which operate (as all agree) by irritation, besides, that the humours before detained and suspended by relaxation, (as in sleep) are now therefore pour'd down in greater quantity by the advanced contraction squeesing them out; as the return of the vigilative contraction after sleep, causes men to be more apt to go to stool upon awaking, or getting up in the morning; which may be well compared (in some measure) to purging, after leaving off the use of opium, since it relaxes as sleep does, and that for a much longer time by a continued use thereof.

IV. Death commonly follows, for all the reasons aforesaid, especially the great and intolerable distresses of soul that

they are under, unless opium be used, which soon sets
them right, or wine (its substitute) so frequently used,
as to continue its cordial pleasure at stomach.[3]

In 1943, C.K. Himmelsbach, Director of Research, U.S. Public Health Service Hospital at Lexington, Kentucky, described well the characteristic withdrawal syndrome associated with withholding derivatives of opium from chronic users.[4] The symptoms included: yawning, lacrimation, rhinorrhea, perspiration, gooseflesh, tremor, dilated pupils, anorexia, nausea, emesis, diarrhea, restlessness, insomnia, weight loss, dehydration, hyperglycemia, elevations of temperature and blood pressure, and alterations of pulse rate. Many of these symptoms were recognized at that time as manifestations of disturbances in the function of the autonomic nervous system.[4] Also recognized at this time was the concept that a negative affective state could accompany these physical signs of opiate withdrawal. Addicts were described as attempting to obtain sufficient drug to "prevent the dysphoria associated with the [opiate] withdrawal syndrome."[5]

Subsequent descriptions of acute opiate withdrawal include a series of symptoms that depend on the type of opiate used, the degree of tolerance (e.g., the amount of opiate used), the time elapsed since the last dose, the interval between doses, and the health and personality of the subject.[6,7] Two types of symptoms have been described: purposive symptoms and nonpurposive symptoms.[6] Purposive symptoms were defined as symptoms which are goal-oriented, highly dependent on the observer and environment, and directed at getting more drug. In contrast, nonpurposive symptoms include those which are not goal-oriented and are relatively independent of the observer, the patient's will, and the environment. The purposive symptoms include such things as complaints, pleas, demands and manipulations, and mimicking of symptoms and are significantly decreased in a hospital setting where they have no consequences.

Both of these types of symptoms also change over time. In the early stages of withdrawal from heroin (6-8 hours after the last dose), purposive behavior is prominent. It peaks at 36-72 hours after the last dose of morphine or heroin. Nonpurposive symptoms including autonomic signs appear at about 8-12 hours after the last dose. There is yawning, sweating and runny nose and eyes (Table 1.1). These mild signs continue increasing in intensity during the first 24 hours and level off. Sometimes at 12-14 hours after the last dose the patient may have a restless sleep called a "yen" which may last for several hours and from which the subject awakens even more uncomfortable.[6] Subsequently, additional nonpurposive symptoms appear which peak at 36-48 hours and continue up to 72 hours. There is pupillary dilation, gooseflesh, hot and cold flashes, loss of appetite, muscle cramps, tremor and insomnia. Autonomic signs include elevations in blood pressure, heart rate, respiratory rate and body temperature accompanied by nausea and vomiting. There are complaints of feeling chilled, alternating with a flushing sensation and excessive sweating. Waves of gooseflesh are prominent, resulting in skin that looks like a plucked turkey, the basis of the expression "cold turkey." Accompanying these symptoms are also the subjective symptoms of aches and pains and general misery such as that associated with a flu-like state. Muscle spasms, uncontrollable muscle twitching and kicking movements are possibly the basis for the expression "kicking the habit." At 24-36 hours, there may be diarrhea and dehydration. The peak of the syndrome appears to be approximately 48-72 hours after the last dose (Table 1.1). Without treatment, the syndrome completes its course in 7-10 days. However, residual subclinical signs may persist for many weeks after withdrawal.[6]

Persistent signs of abstinence in detoxified subjects including hyperthermia, mydriasis, increased blood pressure and increased respiratory rate have been observed to continue for months after opiate withdrawal.[4,8] In subsequent studies, metabolic changes have been reported in an even later stage of protracted abstinence where the direction of the changes is the opposite of the acute signs of abstinence, e.g., hypothermia, miosis, decreased blood pressure, etc.[9] Even more intriguing, a limited exposure to morphine such as a single injection can produce some tolerance to subsequent morphine,[10] and exposure to morphine can dramatically change one's subsequent response to an opiate antagonist,[11] a phenomena sometimes described as acute abstinence.[12] Clearly, opiate dependence represents a long-term perturbation to the central nervous sys-

Table 1.1. Sequence of appearance of some of the abstinence syndrome symptoms

Signs	Approximate Hours After Last Dose	
	Morphine	Heroin and/or Methadone
Craving for drugs, anxiety	6	24
Yawning, perspiration, runny nose, teary eyes	14	34 to 48
Increase in above signs plus pupil dilation, goose bumps (piloerection), tremors (muscle twitches), hot and cold flashes, aching bones and muscles, loss of appetite	16	48 to 72
Increased intensity of above, plus insomnia; raised blood pressure; increased temperature, pulse rate, respiratory rate and depth; restlessness; nausea	24 to 36	
Increased intensity of above, plus curled-up position, vomiting, diarrhea, weight loss, spontaneous ejaculation or orgasm, hemoconcentration, increased blood sugar	36 to 48	

Reproduced with permission from Ray O and Ksir C. Drugs, Society, and Human Behavior, 6th Edition. St. Louis: Mosby, 1993:315.

tem invoking multiple stages of adaptive mechanisms at multiple levels.[13]

Different opiates show similar opiate withdrawal effects that vary in duration and intensity. The withdrawal syndrome from meperidine (Demerol®) usually develops within 3 hours of the last dose, reaches a peak within 8-12 hours and then decreases.[6] In contrast, the abrupt withdrawal from methadone, even after large doses, is slower to develop, less intense and more prolonged. Few or no symptoms are observed for almost 2 days, and peak intensity is reached on the sixth day. These differences in time course and intensity of opiate withdrawal with different opiates speak to the general principle that long-acting drugs produce longer onset,

longer duration and less intense withdrawal than short-acting drugs
(Table 1.2).

The nonpurposive symptoms of opiate withdrawal are formed
not only by the emotional coloring of the physical symptoms and
the direct effects of withdrawal on motivational systems, but also
by associative factors that link these emotional effects to previously neutral stimuli in the environment. Both conditioned positive reinforcement and conditioned negative reinforcement can be
observed in the human situation. One of the earlier experimental
studies on opiate withdrawal described very accurately the changes
in autonomic signs as well as hemodynamic changes in subjects at
the peak of opiate withdrawal (48 hours postopiate).[14] They also
described very carefully the contribution of emotionality to the
nonpurposive symptoms. Even more interesting, this study provided one of the first descriptions of the role of conditioning in
opiate dependence and how stimuli paired with morphine injection could alleviate withdrawal. The following direct quote describes
the signs and symptoms of opiate withdrawal after 48 hours of
abstinence and the conditioned injection effect:

> "Further evidence that the picture of withdrawal symp-
> toms has its basis in an emotional state is the response on
> the part of one of our addicts at the end of a 36 hour
> withdrawal period to the hypodermic injection of sterile

Table 1.2. Withdrawal

	Non-purposive Withdrawal Symptoms (h)	Peak (h)	Time in Which Majority of Symptoms Terminate (d)
Morphine	14-20	36-48	5-10
Heroin	8-12	48-72	5-10
Methadone	36-72 (2nd day)	72-96 (6th day)	14-21
Codeine	24		
Dilaudid	4-5		
Meperidine	4-6	8-12	4-5

Reproduced with permission from Lowinson JH, Ruiz P. Substance Abuse, Clinical Problems
and Perspectives. Baltimore: Williams and Wilkins, 1981:320.

water. Despite his obvious suffering, he immediately went to sleep and slept for eight hours. Addicts frequently speak about the "needle habit," in which the single prick of the needle brings about relief. It is not uncommon for one addict to give another a hypodermic injection of sterile water and the recipient to derive a "kick" and become quiet. On the other hand, it has been our experience just as frequently to have the addict know that he was given a hypodermic injection of sterile water and to have him fail to respond to its effect. Paradoxical as it may seem, we believe that the greater the craving of the addict and the severity of the withdrawal symptoms, the better are the chances of substituting a hypodermic injection of sterile water to obtain temporary relief."[15]

Subsequent studies of this phenomena have called these individuals "needle freaks" where at least part of the relief and pleasure they obtain from injecting the drug is the result of a conditioned positive response to the injection procedure associated with heroin use.[15,16] Indeed, in an experimental situation under double-blind conditions, subjects were administered an opiate antagonist and then allowed to self-administer vehicle or opiate. All of the self-injections were rated as pleasurable at first, and after 3-5 injections the subjects reported neutral effects.[15,16]

That conditioned negative reinforcement can contribute to the manifestations of opiate withdrawal is now well documented and has been demonstrated experimentally. O'Brien in the following direct quote describes the experience of an opiate addict upon returning to an environment where he had previously experienced opiate withdrawal.[17]

"For example, one patient who was slowly detoxified after methadone maintenance went to visit relatives in Los Angeles after receiving his last dose. Since he knew that he would be away from the clinic in Philadelphia for three weeks, he saved one take-home bottle of methadone in case he got sick while in California. To his surprise, he felt no sickness while in this new environment and never even thought about the bottle of methadone in his suitcase. He felt healthy over the three-week, drug-free period, but as soon as he arrived in the Philadelphia airport, he began to experience craving. By the time he reached his home, there was yawning and tearing. He immediately took the methadone he had been saving and felt relieved, but the symptoms recurred the next day. After three weeks of being symptom-free in Los Angeles, he experienced regular withdrawal in Philadelphia."[17]

This conditioned withdrawal was then experimentally induced. Methadone-maintained individual volunteers were subjected to repeated episodes of precipitated opiate withdrawal by a very small dose of naloxone (0.1 mg IM) in the context of a tone and peppermint smell in a particular environment. This dose of naloxone elicited tearing, rhinorrhea, yawning, decreased skin temperature, increased respiratory rate and subjective feelings of drug sickness and craving. Subsequently, injection of vehicle (physiological saline) accompanied by the peppermint smell and tone elicited reliable signs and symptoms of opiate withdrawal that were similar to the precipitated withdrawal, though less severe.[18]

Thus, there is a rich history of opiate withdrawal that has accurately described its occurrence and nature for several hundred years. More recent descriptions have distinguished different aspects of opiate withdrawal, e.g., purposive (motivational) versus nonpurposive (physical) symptoms that provide a framework for understanding the mechanisms of opiate withdrawal. In addition, the powerful nature of the effects of opiate withdrawal is shown by the more recent demonstrations of conditioned withdrawal effects. Animal models exist for all aspects of opiate withdrawal and these animal models are critical to the study of the neurobiology of opiate withdrawal described in the subsequent chapters.

REFERENCES

1. Macht DI. The history of opium and some of its preparation and alkaloids. J Am Med Assoc 1915; 64:477-481.
2. Latham RG. The Works of Thomas Sydenham, M.D. London: C.J. Adlard Printers, 1848.

3. Jones JR. The Mysteries of Opium Revealed. London: Richard Smith at the Angel and Bible without Temple-Bar, 1700.
4. Himmelsbach CK. Symposium: Can the euphoric, analgetic, and physical dependence effects of drugs be separated? IV. With reference to physical dependence. Fed Proc 1943; 2:201-203.
5. Reichard JD. Symposium: Can the euphoric, analgetic and physical dependence effects of drugs be separated? I. With reference to euphoria. Fed Proc 1943; 2:188-191.
6. Council Reports. Treatment of morphine-type dependence by withdrawal methods. J Am Med Assoc 1972; 219:1611-1615.
7. Gelenberg AJ, Bassuk EL, Schoonover SC. The Practitioner's Guide to Psychoactive Drugs. 3rd ed. New York: Plenum Publishing Corp., 1991.
8. Himmelsbach CK. Clinical studies of drug addiction: Physical dependence, withdrawal and recovery. Arch Intern Med 1942; 69:766-772.
9. Martin WR, Jasinski DR. Physiological parameters of morphine dependence in man—Tolerance, early abstinence, protracted abstinence. J Psychiatr Res 1969; 7:9-17.
10. Cochin J, Kornetsky C. Development and loss of tolerance to morphine in the rat after single and multiple injections. J Pharmacol Exp Ther 1964; 145:1-10.
11. Crowley TJ, Wagner JE, Zerbe G. Naltrexone-induced dysphoria in former opioid addicts. Am J Psychiatry 1985; 142:1081-1084.
12. Heishman SJ, Stitzer ML, Bigelow GE et al. Acute opioid physical dependence in humans: Effect of varying the morphine-naloxone interval. J Pharmacol Exp Ther 1989; 250:485-491.
13. Koob GF, Bloom FE. Cellular and molecular mechanisms of drug dependence. Science 1988; 242:715-723.
14. Light AB, Torrance EG. Opium addiction. VI. The effects of abrupt withdrawal followed by administration of morphine in human addicts, with special reference to the composition of the blood, the circulation and the metabolism. Arch Intern Med 1929; 44:1-16.
15. O'Brien CP. "Needle freaks:" Psychological dependence on shooting up. In: Medical World News, Psychiatry Annual. New York: McGraw Hill, 1974.
16. Meyer RE, Mirin SM. The Heroin Stimulus: Implications for a Theory of Addiction. New York: Plenum Press, 1979.
17. O'Brien CP, Ehrman RN, Ternes JM. Classical conditioning in human opioid dependence. In: Goldberg SR, Stolerman IP, eds. Behavioral Analysis of Drug Dependence. London: Academic Press, 1986:329-356.
18. O'Brien CP, Jesta J, O'Brien TJ et al. Conditioned narcotic withdrawal in humans. Science 1977; 195:1000-1002.

CHAPTER 2

ANIMAL MODELS OF OPIATE DEPENDENCE

PROCEDURE USED TO INDUCE OPIATE DEPENDENCE

Endogenous opioid peptides exert a wide range of central and peripheral effects. It was thought that tolerance to opiates could be assessed for any of its measurable actions. However, tolerance develops to many different effects of morphine, to different degrees and at different rates. Moreover, some effects seem to be unchanged while others increase after repeated opiate administration. Thus, these adaptive mechanisms, which develop for each morphine effect, must not have absolute common bases. They must depend upon the interaction between the overstimulation of opioid receptors by opiates and the complex neuronal circuitries responsible for the physiological effects. It is important to emphasize that these adaptive processes are mediated through physiological feedback mechanisms. Following the repeated exposure to the drug, their activities will increase out of the physiological range, and this situation will become progressively permanent and will establish a new artificial homeostatic equilibrium of the "milieu interieur," in which the opiate will exert a controlling role in the sense that the permanent stimulation of opiate receptors is now needed. In opiate-addicted subjects, abstinence of the drug will disrupt this artificial homeostatic state triggering physiological, behavioral and psychological effects. Together, these symptoms will define opiate dependence. Thus, one must consider that when a subject is tolerant or sensitized to a given drug effect, the subject is dependent on the drug as a whole.

In order to study the development of these adaptive processes, several animal models of opiate-induced dependence are available. Since it appears that the degree of tolerance developed is directly related to the duration of exposure to the compound, in terms of both dose and kinetics, methods for maintaining optimal exposure have followed two basic strategies: the multiple injection (or intake) procedure and continuous exposure. However, as we will see, some manifestations of opiate dependence can be detected even after a single injection of a high dose of opiate. As we will see, the choice of these methods for induction of opiate dependence is also guided by the type of abstinence state one wants to produce, either pharmacologically- or spontaneously-induced. For each case we will give an example of the experimental protocols currently used.

INDUCTION OF MORPHINE DEPENDENCE BY ORAL INTAKE OF THE DRUG

Oral intake of opiate drugs may be used to produce opiate dependence only if the drugs used are orally active. Morphine sulfate, which is usually employed to produce such effects, has a poor absorption from the gastrointestinal tract, and for this reason several weeks of treatment with high doses of morphine are needed to induce a robust opiate dependence.

Morphine in food

Morphine can be added to daily food. The concentration of morphine (base) in food is increased weekly from 0.5 mg/g food the first week to 2 mg/g food after the third week. During the first 2 days, animals were food-deprived in order to force consumption of the morphine-food mix during the following days. During the first week, a delay in the increase of body weight occurs, due to the low food intake probably caused by the aversion to the food. During the following weeks, body weight increase is similar to that of control animals. After the third week, food-morphine mix intake is about 25 g, corresponding to 50 mg of morphine base by rat or 160 mg/kg body weight per day. This method allows one to maintain for weeks a plasma concentration of 1 mg/l.[1,2]

Morphine in water

Several protocols are available. A classic one is as follows: morphine-drinking rats are provided with water bottles containing a solution of 0.1 mg/ml of morphine on the first day. The concentration of the solution is then increased to 0.25 mg/ml on the sixth day, and to 0.5 mg/ml on the eleventh day. Rats are given 5 minute access to their water bottles every 6 hours. The beginning and end of each access period is signaled by a 10 second tone. In some studies a saccharin-water solution (0.2 mg/ml) has been used to overcome the bitterness of morphine. After 16 days on the schedule of limited access to the fluid, volumes of fluids consumed by the control rats and morphine-drinking rats are similar—100 ml/kg of body weight—which corresponds to an average of 53 mg/kg/day of morphine intake. The only consistently obvious difference between groups is a slight decrease in the rate of weight gain by the morphine drinkers. At least 3-4 weeks of this regimen is needed in order to produce a maximal opiate dependence as evidenced by the intensity of the naloxone-precipitated withdrawal score. Then, a constant plasma concentration of morphine of 0.2 mg/l of plasma was reached.[3]

INDUCTION OF OPIATE DEPENDENCE
BY MULTIPLE INJECTIONS OF MORPHINE

In general, a high degree of dependence is rapidly attainable after repeated injections of high doses of morphine; however, as will be seen later, some signs of an acute abstinence can be detected after a single injection of a relatively high dose of opiates. The duration of the treatment depends on the dose used. Classically, morphine dependence can be induced in rats by intraperitoneal injections of morphine twice a day for 10 days according to the following design: 5 mg/kg the first day, 10 mg/kg the second, and then increasing by 10 mg/kg per day to reach a dose of 90 mg/kg per injection on the tenth day. Injections are delivered at 08:00 and 20:00. For the first 4 days the injection volume was 1 ml/kg; for the following days it was increased to 2 ml/kg. Control rats receive the same injections except that morphine was omitted. While the concentration of morphine follows an up-and-down pattern according to the time elapsed after the last injection, this procedure resembles human drug intake patterns and is a rapid and suitable method to analyze the evolution of spontaneous morphine withdrawal induced by the abstinence of the drug and to study protracted effects of opiate dependence[4] (Stinus et al, 1996, unpublished).

Opiate dependence can be also induced by repeated intravenous injections of either morphine or methadone. Such a schedule of injections yields interinjection intervals and daily drug intakes similar to those obtained in dependent self-administering rats. The initial dose of morphine is 1.25 mg/kg/2 hours for 24 hours, which is then increased on successive days to 2.5, 5 and 10 mg/kg/2 hours. The initial dose of methadone is 0.25 mg/kg/2 hours for 24 hours, which is increased on successive days to 0.5, 1 and 2 mg/kg/2 hours.[5,6]

INDUCTION OF OPIATE DEPENDENCE BY CONTINUOUS EXPOSURE TO MORPHINE

Continuous exposure to morphine can be achieved by either subcutaneous implantation of slow-release morphine pellets or osmotic minipumps (Alzet) filled with opiates which will continuously release the drug for 1 or 2 weeks.

Subcutaneous implantation of morphine pellets

The subcutaneous implantation of slow-release, morphine-containing pellets is a rapid and reliable method to produce opiate dependence. Long-lasting morphine pellets are provided by the National Institute on Drug Abuse (NIDA, USA). Each morphine pellet contains 75 mg morphine base, 69.27 mg Avicel PH-102, 1.5 mg magnesium stearate NF, 1.5 mg colloidal silicon dioxide NF and 1.75 mg purified water USP; placebo pellets contain no morphine, 150 mg Avicel PH-102, 1.5 mg magnesium stearate NF, 1.5 mg colloidal silicon dioxide NF and 1.75 mg purified water USP. Under light anesthesia (halothane/air 4/100 V/V for 30 seconds), two 75 mg morphine-containing pellets are implanted subcutaneously (low back). Plasma concentration of morphine is maintained constant for at least 12 days (0.1-0.2 mg/l of plasma). Usually, opiate withdrawal is induced by the injection of naloxone

(1 mg/kg subcutaneously). The first symptoms of naloxone-induced opiate withdrawal are observed as early as 3 hours postimplantation, and a full abstinence syndrome is recorded after the first day of opiate exposure (Fig. 2.1 and Table 2.1). This situation remains permanent for 15 days after which dependence to opiates decreases as the content of the morphine in pellets is exhausted. The efficacy of this method is due to the maintenance of a constant level of morphine in the blood.[7,8] Similar results were obtained with different pellet formulations.[9,10]

Table 2.1. The Gellert-Holtzman rating score

Sign	Weighting Factor
Graded Signs	
Weight loss in 2-1/2 hours (each 1% above the weight lost by control rats)	1
No. of escape attempts	
2-4	1
5-9	2
10 or more	3
No. of abdominal contractions (each one)	2
No. of wet dog shakes	
1-2	2
3 or more	4
Checked Signs	
Diarrhea	2
Facial fasciculations or teeth chattering	2
Swallowing	2
Profuse salivation	7
Chromodacryorrhea	5
Ptosis	2
Abnormal posture	3
Erection, ejaculation or genital grooming	3
Irritability	3

Gellert-Holtzman rating score. This scale includes graded as well as checked signs. Reproduced with permission from Gellert VF, Holtzman SG, J Pharmacol Exp Ther 1978; 205:536-546.

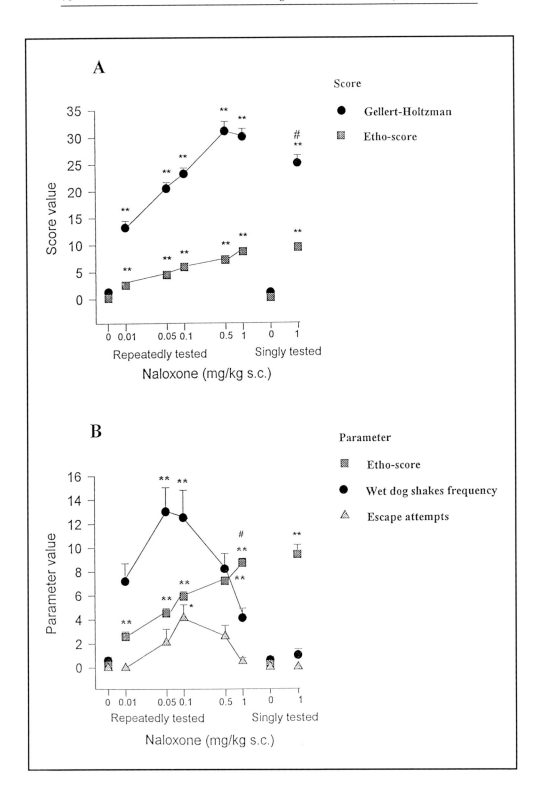

Subcutaneous implantation of osmotic minipumps

While osmotic minipumps can be used for subcutaneous release of opiates, they are a perfectly reliable tool to introduce drugs directly into the intracerebroventricular (ICV) space. Specific agonists or antagonists of opiate receptors and their respective control solutions can be perfused ICV into the rat brain using osmotic minipumps (Model 2001, Alzet-Alza Corp., Palo Alto, CA) with a flow rate of 1 μl/hour and a reservoir volume sufficient for 7 days. The minipump with the connecting polyethylene tube is prefilled with drug or vehicle solution and then implanted subcutaneously. The polyethylene tube is connected to a stainless steel cannula guide stereotaxically implanted ICV.[11]

MODELS TO EVALUATE OPIATE DEPENDENCE

INDUCTION OF OPIATE ABSTINENCE

In opiate-dependent rats, abstinence to the drug can be triggered either spontaneously by the omission of the drug treatment or pharmacologically by the blockade of opiate receptors induced by administration of an opiate receptor antagonist.

Spontaneous withdrawal will be induced by the discontinuation of the opiate availability, either by the reinstatement of normal food and water intake when the drug was consumed orally or by cessation of injections when injected (intraperitoneally or intravenously), or by removal of morphine pellets in morphine-pelleted rats. However, this last method needs a second surgical procedure which could interfere with the kinetics of opiate abstinence.

*Fig. 2.1 (opposite). Intensity of naloxone-induced withdrawal syndrome (dose response) and comparison of its evaluation by either the Gellert-Holtzman or the etho-score scales. Morphine dependence was induced by subcutaneous implantation of two morphine pellets (2 x 75 mg, NIDA). Opiate withdrawal was induced after either repeated (once daily in random order) or single (1 mg/kg subcutaneously) tests. (A) Values of the Gellert-Holtzman score and etho-score. (B) Values of etho-score, wet-dog shakes frequency and escape attempts. Repeatedly and singly tested groups are separately represented along the horizontal axes. MEAN ± SEM; *p<0.05, **p<0.01 vs. control group; #p<0.05 vs. 1 mg/kg naloxone in the repeatedly tested group. Reproduced with permission from Espejo EF et al, Psychopharmacology 1995; 122:122-130.*

Pharmacologically-induced opiate withdrawal is generally produced by subcutaneous injection of naloxone in rats rendered dependent by any of the procedures described above. However, the most reliable experimental approach to study naloxone-precipitated opiate withdrawal is the pellet implantation method. A poor dose-response relationship with increasing naloxone efficacy dose ranges of 0.01-10 mg/kg subcutaneously has been reported, presumably due to the fact that naloxone is a powerful opiate antagonist.[12] However, when full opiate dependence has been achieved 3 days after subcutaneous implantation of two morphine pellets (75 mg x 2), doses of 0.1-1 mg/kg are sufficient to induce a full somatic withdrawal syndrome, while these doses are without effect in placebo-pelleted rats.[7,13] Moreover, as one will observe below, all behavioral signs of opiate abstinence can be precipitated by naloxone doses as low as 0.03 mg/kg subcutaneously.[13]

EVALUATION OF SOMATIC INDICES OF OPIATE DEPENDENCE

The evaluation of somatic signs of withdrawal is generally performed by scoring several physical signs for 10 minutes, either following the injection of an opiate receptor antagonist when opiate withdrawal is pharmacologically triggered[3,7-9,13-15] or every 6 or 9 hours for 3-5 days when spontaneous abstinence is produced.[4] A weighted scale of Gellert and Holtzman[3] can be used as an overall index of withdrawal intensity (Table 2.1). This scale consists of graded signs of weight loss (measured 2.5 hours after the naloxone injection), number of escape attempts, number of wet dog shakes, instances of abdominal constrictions, and checked signs (simply scored as present or absent) including diarrhea, facial fasciculations/teeth chattering, swallowing movements, profuse salivation, chromodacryorrhea, ptosis, abnormal posture, penile grooming/erection/ejaculation, and irritability upon handling. There is a close similarity between somatic signs of opiate withdrawal in animals and those observed in human heroin addicts during acute opiate abstinence.[16] In rats, some of these signs become progressively more pronounced when dependence gets stronger or the dose of opiate receptor antagonist is increased (teeth chattering, weight loss). In contrast, other signs showed a maximal frequency at the lower degree of dependence or after administration of the lower doses of naloxone and decreased or even disappeared when the degree of dependence or the dose of naloxone was further increased (i.e., wet dog shakes, jumps).[3,7-9,13] If naloxone (1 mg/kg subcutaneously) is injected as soon as 3 hours following implantation of two morphine pellets, the following signs are repeatedly observed: facial fasciculations and teeth chattering, swallowing movements, irritability and vocalizations when handled, abnormal postures, and weight loss. If naloxone is injected at 12 hours postimplantation, in addition to these signs, wet dog shakes, ptosis and penile erection with or without ejaculation can also be recorded. A full withdrawal syndrome was registered as soon as 24 hours and remained stable for 12 days.[7,13,14] It is interesting to emphasize that the rats showed naloxone-induced abstinence signs 3 hours after pellet implantation while the rats still exhibited full analgesia.[14]

Whereas the Gellert and Holtzman[3] scale for somatic signs of withdrawal has been a useful and reliable approach in order to quantify opiate abstinence, the validity of the selection criteria of signs and scores has never been confronted with an ethological analysis. Ethopharmacological analysis of naloxone-precipitated morphine withdrawal syndrome using a multivariate cluster analysis based on similarity values between patterns gives a more precise overview[15] (Fig. 2.1). In placebo-pelleted rats, only two clear-cut categories of patterns are identified, "exploration patterns" comprising immobile sniffing and walk-sniffing and "self-care patterns" made up of face-washing and self-grooming. Following naloxone treatment of morphine-pelleted rats, in addition to the above categories which are maintained, two new categories emerged: "writhing behavior," which is composed of writhing postures and attenuated gait, and "escape" made up of jumping and leaning postures. From this study, a simple, newly developed rating score was defined based on mastication (teeth chattering) and weight loss. This "etho-score" changes in a dose-dependent fashion (from 0.01 to 1 mg/kg subcutaneously) and is little affected by learning, which allows repeated measures on a given subject.

Etho-score = (MF/10) + WL. The first component of the formula is a behavioral variable based on mastication frequency (MF; each burst of mastication was qualified as 1 regardless of its duration). The second component is a physical factor based on weight loss (WL; each 1% body weight loss during the 2 hours following naloxone injection is quantified as 1).[15]

EVALUATION OF BEHAVIORAL EFFECTS OF OPIATE WITHDRAWAL

Clinical evidence indicates that the affective signs of opiate abstinence may be more relevant to drug craving and relapse to compulsive drug use than the somatic signs of withdrawal.[17,18] Thus, animal models of the affective aspects of opiate withdrawal are important tools for understanding the neurobiological bases of opiate dependence and for development of effective strategies to alleviate acute abstinence syndrome, reduce drug craving and prevent relapse. We will review the behavioral alterations which have been hypothesized to serve as measures of the affective symptoms of acute opiate withdrawal.

Spontaneous locomotor activity recording

Locomotor activity of rats undergoing acute opiate abstinence can be measured for long periods of time in rectangular cages which have two infrared beams across the long axis of the cage 2 cm above the floor. Total photocell beam interruptions and crossovers are automatically recorded. If food and water are available in the cage, this procedure can be applied for weeks[13,19] (Stinus et al, 1996, unpublished).

Naloxone-induced opiate withdrawal following morphine pellet implantation

During the habituation period prior to the naloxone injection, morphine-dependent rats are more active than their respective controls. A dose as little as 0.01 mg/kg of naloxone reliably elicits decreases in spontaneous locomotor activity in opiate-dependent rats while a dose of 0.1 mg is needed to induce similar effects in control rats.[13]

Spontaneous opiate withdrawal following escalating doses of morphine for 10 days

Continuous quantitative evaluation of spontaneous opiate withdrawal can be performed by continuous recording of locomotor activity for 11 days (Fig. 2.2). While control rats displayed a typical locomotor activity pattern characterized by nocturnal hyperactivity which is markedly reduced during the light phase, opiate-abstinent rats developed a constant motor activity which is observed during the first 3 or 4 postinjection days. Although morphine-abstinent rats slowly resumed a normal circadian cycle after the fourth day, long-term effects are revealed by the permanent motor instability recorded during both the light and dark phases (Stinus et al, 1996, unpublished). These early disturbances paralleled the somatic and behavioral symptoms of withdrawal in morphine-dependent rats.[19-21] Similar results have been also shown by other studies using shorter recording periods.[1,2,22,23]

DISRUPTION OF OPERANT RESPONDING FOR FOOD

This experimental procedure is based on opiate withdrawal-induced disruption of an operant conditioning for food. Rats were trained to lever-press in operant chambers for 45 mg food pellets on a continuous reinforcement fixed ratio (FR-1) schedule (Fig. 2.3). Subsequently, the FR schedule of reinforcement was gradually increased to 15. Then rats responded on an FR-15 schedule during 30 minute sessions until a stable rate of responding was achieved. Rats were then implanted with placebo or morphine (75 mg x 2) pellets and trained again for 4 days. On the final testing day after a 10 minute session, control and morphine-dependent rats received a subcutaneous injection of solvent or different doses of naloxone. Naloxone reduced responding in morphine-pelleted rats with a near-complete suppression by a 0.03 mg/kg dose, while responding was unaffected in placebo pellet controls.[13] Similar results were triggered by intracerebral injection of very small amounts (4 ng) of methylnaloxonium, an opiate receptor antagonist, in morphine-dependent rats, particularly in the nucleus accumbens which is one of the key limbic structures for the reinforcing effects of opiates.[24]

INTRACRANIAL SELF-STIMULATION

The purpose of this approach is to evaluate the excitability of the reward system by means of implanted electrodes in the medial forebrain bundle.[25,26] The procedure is a modification of the

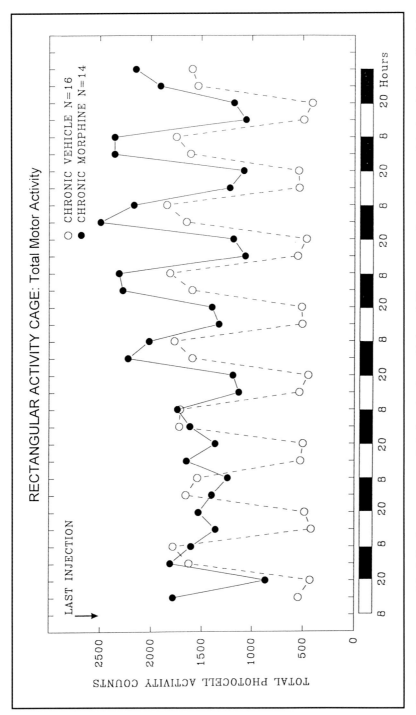

Fig. 2.2. Locomotor activity following spontaneously induced opiate withdrawal. Time course of total motor activity (total photocell activity counts) recorded in rectangular activity cages during 8 days following opiate withdrawal. Chronic morphine-treated rats (n = 14) received twice daily for 10 days increasing doses of morphine (up to 90 mg/kg intraperitoneally) (black circles and solid lines). Chronic vehicle group (n = 16) received the same treatment except that the drug was omitted (white circles and dotted lines). Maximal and minimal standard deviation to the mean (±SEM) were 8% and 12% of activity values. Reproduced with permission from Stinus L. In: Stefanis C, Hippius H, eds. Psychiatry in Progress: Research in Addiction, Vol. 2. Seattle: Hogrefe and Huber Publishing, 1995:1-21.

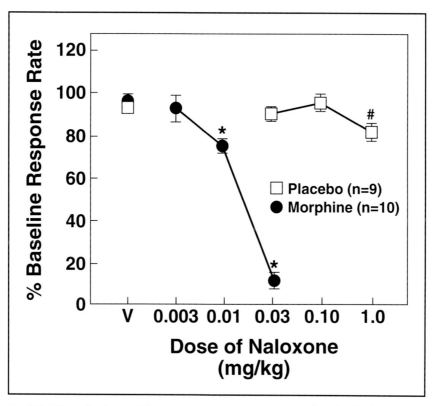

Fig. 2.3. Effect of naloxone (dose response) on operant responding for food. Rats were trained under a FR-15 schedule (rats must press 15 times on the lever in order to obtain a food pellet) in placebo-pelleted and morphine-pelleted rats (two placebo or two 75-mg morphine pellets, NIDA). The minimum dose of naloxone that suppressed responding in placebo-pelleted rats was 1 mg/kg (#p<0.05 vs. vehicle). In morphine-pelleted rats, the minimal effective dose was 0.01 mg/kg subcutaneously of naloxone; a dose of 0.03 mg/kg suppressed responding almost entirely (*p<0.05 vs. V). Reproduced with permission from Schulteis G et al, J Pharmacol Exp Ther 1994; 271:1391-1398.

Kornetsky and Esposito[27] discrete-trial current threshold procedure. After acquisition of operant responding for intracranial self-stimulation (ICSS) and establishment of stable baseline thresholds, the electrical stimulation threshold for ICSS was determined in placebo and morphine pellet-implanted rats, both after receiving solvent or naloxone subcutaneously.[13] To start each trial, a rat received a noncontingent electrical stimulus. A correct response was recorded if a rat rotated a wheel manipulandum at least one-quarter turn within 7.5 seconds of the noncontingent electrical stimulus; each correct response produced a contingent stimulus identical in all parameters to the noncontingent stimulus. Stimulus intensities varied with a step size of 5 μg according to the method of limits. A given stimulus intensity was presented three times within each series. Threshold was defined for each series as the midpoint between the current intensity level at which at least two correct responses occurred and that level at which fewer than two responses occurred. As already observed,[28] in placebo-pelleted rats administration of naloxone at doses up to 1 mg/kg was without significant effect on ICSS threshold. However, in morphine-dependent rats, naloxone induced a significant dose-dependent elevation in ICSS thresholds with a significant effect with doses as low as 0.03 mg/kg (165% of baseline).[13]

SLEEP DISORDERS AND SPONTANEOUS OPIATE WITHDRAWAL

Abstinence from morphine induced by interruption of its injection following escalating doses twice daily for 10 days shows profound modifications of waking (W), nonrapid eye movement sleep (NREMS) and rapid eye movement sleep (REMS) automatically detected from an 11-day period of electrocorticogram recording (Fig. 2.4). The disruption of the circadian locomotor activity rhythm during the first 4 postinjection days (see above) was associated with an important insomnia as revealed by the drastic reduction of overall REMS and NREMS and the increase of W. The natural rhythm reappeared at the end of the fourth day and restarted slowly from then on. However, the analysis of the percentage of REMS over the total sleeping time (%REMS/TST) reveals long-term perturbations induced by the experience of opiate dependence and abstinence. In vehicle-treated rats, we observed a regular oscillation of %REMS/TST values from a peak during the light phase (19.5%) and a minimal value during the night (9.4%). In contrast, the circadian evolution of %REMS/TST was disrupted during the 11 days of recording following morphine abstinence (Stinus et al, 1996, unpublished). Using a variety of different techniques for establishment of morphine dependence, similar sleep disorders have already been reported.[29-31] In addition, in some studies a short-lived REMS rebound has been detected during the third or fourth day postabstinence.[31,32]

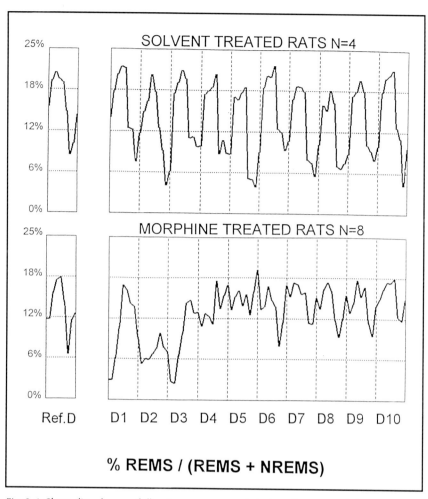

Fig. 2.4. Sleep disturbances following spontaneously induced opiate withdrawal. Opiate dependence was induced by injection of increasing doses of morphine. Time course of REMS in percent of total sleep time (REMS + NREMS) (% REMS / REMS + NREMS) during first, a reference day (Ref. D) recorded just before the pharmacological treatment, and during the first 10 days which followed abstinence (day 1 to day 10). Chronic morphine-treated rats received twice a day for 10 days increasing doses of morphine (up to 90 mg/kg intraperitoneally) (lower panel, n = 8). Chronic vehicle group received the same treatment except that the drug was omitted (upper panel, n = 4). In order to clarify data presentation, SEM was omitted; at the most it represented 2.2 %REMS, rapid eye movement sleep; NREMS, nonrapid eye movement sleep.

CONDITIONED OPIATE WITHDRAWAL

Significant clinical evidence suggests that individuals experiencing drug withdrawal can become conditioned to environmental situations. Previously neutral stimuli can elicit many of the symptoms of opiate abstinence if paired with the withdrawal state, and this conditioned withdrawal may have motivational significance in drug dependence.[33,34] The following paragraphs will present two experimental schedules for quantifiable measurement of conditioned opiate withdrawal in the rat.

Conditioned place aversion

Pharmacologically-precipitated opiate withdrawal induces conditioned place aversion which can be seen at doses of opiate antagonists that produce few if any overt somatic signs of withdrawal.[35-37] Briefly, the conditioned place aversion apparatus used to induce a reliable aversion[37-39] consists of three rectangular boxes (40 x 33 x 34 cm) spaced at 120° angles and all accessible from a triangular central compartment. Distinctive visual, tactile and olfactory cues distinguish the three compartments. Each compartment is equipped with photocells to allow automatic detection and recording with a computer of an animal's position at all times. The apparatus is located in a sound-attenuated testing room, with white noise (75 db) to further mask external noise, and illuminated by three 15 W red lights located 1.5 meters above each compartment. The experimental protocol consists of three distinct phases: a preconditioning phase, a conditioning phase and a testing phase.

In the preconditioning phase (3 days after the implantation of two pellets of either placebo or morphine 75 mg), animals were placed in the central triangular compartment and allowed to freely explore the apparatus for 20 minutes. For each rat, the two compartments with the most similar time allotments were randomly paired either with a dose of naloxone (0.002-0.12 mg/kg subcutaneously) or vehicle (Table 2.2). The third compartment was not paired with an injection. Importantly, after the compartment assignments were completed, there were no significant differences between time spent in the naloxone-paired (mean = 409 seconds), vehicle-paired (mean = 391 seconds) or neutral (mean = 392 seconds) compartments during the preconditioning phase. This is an important step in the experimental procedure which avoids any preference bias prior to conditioning.

In the conditioning phase, rats received injections of vehicle on days 4, 6 and 8 postpellet implantation prior to being con-

Table 2.2. Conditioned place aversions as a function of naloxone dose in morphine-pelleted rats

	Time Spent in Naloxone-Paired Compartment (sec)[a]	
	Preconditioning Phase	Testing Phase
Dose of Naloxone (mg/kg)		
0.002 (n = 10)	374 ± 20	371 ± 48
0.004 (n = 10)	410 ± 29	308 ± 28[*]
0.008 (n = 8)	381 ± 22	198 ± 24[*]
0.03 (n = 7)	400 ± 27	194 ± 33[*]
0.06 (n = 5)	419 ± 48	168 ± 51[*]
0.12 (n = 5)	449 ± 34	181 ± 41[*]

[a]Data expressed as mean ± SEM

[*]$p < 0.05$ vs. time in naloxone-paired side during preconditioning phase

Naloxone-induced conditioned place aversion: A dose response study. Conditioned place aversion was evaluated in a three-compartment testing apparatus, and each compartment could be differentiated by the rat by the use of distinctive cues. One of these compartments was associated three times to naloxone-induced withdrawal. Time spent in the naloxone-paired compartment before conditioning and after conditioning is reported ([*]$p < 0.05$ vs. time in naloxone-paired site during preconditioning phase). Morphine dependence was induced by subcutaneous implantation of two morphine pellets (2 x 75 mg, NIDA).

Reproduced with permission from Schulteis G et al, J Pharmacol Exp Ther 1994; 271:1391-1398.

fined to their preselected, vehicle-paired compartment for 20 minutes. On days 5, 7 and 9 post-pellet implantation, rats received one of several doses of naloxone immediately prior to confinement in the naloxone-paired compartment for 20 minutes.

The testing phase consisted of 20 minutes free exploration of the entire apparatus on day 10 postpellet implantation. The difference in time spent on the naloxone-paired side during the testing phase and the time spent in the same compartment during the preconditioning phase served as an index of place aversion. In morphine-pelleted rats, naloxone dose-dependently produced a conditioned place aversion which was observed with a dose of naloxone as low as 0.004 mg/kg (-102 seconds) (Table 2.2) and which was maximum for doses up to 0.008 mg/kg (-206 seconds). Moreover, for these naloxone doses no somatic withdrawal signs could be detected. In placebo-pelleted rats, doses of naloxone which produced profound place aversions in morphine-dependent rats had no effect on time spent in the naloxone-paired compartment.

Operant conditioning and conditioned opiate withdrawal

Operant conditioning for food can be used to produce a rapid and quantifiable measure of conditioned opiate withdrawal.[40] After rats were trained to lever-press for food reinforcement on a FR-15 schedule, they were implanted with two subcutaneous 75 mg morphine pellets and allocated into three groups (paired, unpaired and control). The paired group received four naloxone injections (0.025 mg/kg subcutaneously) in the operant chamber paired with a distinctive tone and smell. The unpaired group was also exposed to the tone and smell in the chambers on four occasions, but received the naloxone injections in the home cage. The saline control animals were never exposed to naloxone or the tone and smell. On the test day, the animals were tested on a FR-15 schedule for 30 minutes. All rats were exposed to the tone and smell and injected with saline 10 minutes after the start of the test. The paired group showed a significant reduction in operant responding in response to the tone and smell when compared either with the other two groups or to their own response rates on the previous day (Fig. 2.5). In a second experiment, in order to test for conditioned withdrawal in postdependent rats, the paired and unpaired groups were again challenged with the tone and smell and saline injection 1 month after removal of the morphine pellets. Again, the paired group showed a significant disruption of response. These results suggest that the conditioned stimulus-acquired significant behavior-disruptive properties manifest even in the absence of opiate receptor occupancy.

OPIATE PHYSICAL DEPENDENCE DEVELOPMENT: EFFECTS OF SINGLE VERSUS REPEATED MORPHINE TREATMENTS

Pharmacologically-precipitated opiate withdrawal signs have been reported in humans and in animals after a single exposure to opiate agonist. These symptoms have been named acute opiate physical dependence.[41] Forty-five minutes after a single injection of morphine in nondependent male opiate users while agonist effects are clearly observed, naloxone reversed these effects and simultaneously precipitated subjective symptoms and observer-rated signs of opiate withdrawal.[41] More intense signs were seen after

Fig. 2.5. Conditioned withdrawal. Rats were trained on operant responding for food under a FR-15 schedule. Morphine dependence was induced by implantation of two morphine pellets (2 x 75 mg, NIDA). The paired group (solid circles) had four previous experiences during which naloxone injection (0.25 mg/kg subcutaneously) was paired in the operant chamber with a distinctive tone and smell. The unpaired group (solid triangles) also had four previous experiences of naloxone-induced opiate withdrawal but was never paired to tone and smell. The saline control group (solid squares) had never experienced naloxone-induced opiate withdrawal. On the test day, all rats

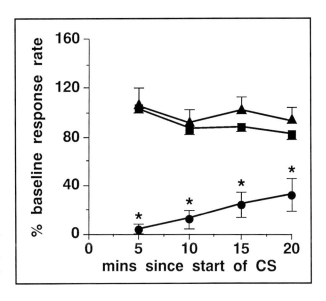

were exposed to the tone and smell and injected with saline. Values are mean ± SEM percentage of baseline rate of lever-pressing/minute. Mean ± SEM pretreatment baseline rates on the test day were as follows: paired group = 60.0 ± 8.4; unpaired group = 74.7 ± 8.1; saline controls = 95.1 ± 8.7 lever-presses/minute. * indicates results significantly different from the unpaired group and saline controls (p<0.05). Reproduced with permission from Baldwin HA, Koob GF, Neuropsychopharmacology 1993; 8:15-21.

repeated morphine treatment.[42] Similarly, while naloxone did not modify tail-flick reflex in lightly anesthetized rats, after a single dose of morphine, naloxone not only reduced morphine-induced analgesia but also induced hyperalgesia, the magnitude of which was correlated to the morphine dose.[43] These acute withdrawal signs can also be observed without any opiate antagonist administration since postencounter or morphine-induced analgesia were followed by a short-lasting hyperalgesia in mice.[44] In all studies cited until now, pharmacological treatment consisted of high doses of either single or repeated administration of opiates which induced a high incidence of opiate abstinence; however, a substantial subgroup of heroin addicts are able to use opioids regularly while maintaining relatively low levels of physical dependence.[45]

PROTRACTED EFFECTS OF OPIATE ABSTINENCE

In opiate-dependent subjects there are many physiological measures that require several months following withdrawal to return to normal. Following opiate abstinence, protracted effects of morphine dependence were revealed by the increase of spontaneous motor activities, both during day and night and by the loss of %REMS/total sleep circadian rhythm (Stinus et al, 1996, unpublished). Protracted effects of morphine intoxication have also been reported in several studies. From day 4 to day 63 postmorphine treatment, rats develop an increased respiratory and metabolic rate and body temperature as well as a decreased fluid intake.[20] Postdependent animals remained tolerant to the depressant effect of high doses of morphine. When challenged with morphine after 15 days and up to 1 year of morphine abstinence, early EEG and behavioral stupor were reduced, while subsequent EEG and behavioral arousal were increased when compared to chronic saline-treated rats.[23,32,46,47] While naloxone has no effect on locomotor activity of control rats, it has a depressant effect in both dependent and postdependent rats.[23] Once made morphine-dependent, rats spontaneously show intense aggression upon grouping, even 30 days after complete abstinence, which was blocked by low doses of morphine and dependent upon dopaminergic supersensitivity.[48,49] Finally, the acquisition of reference and working memories was impaired in a Y-maze and radial maze up to 9 months after chronic morphine treatment,[21,50] suggesting the possibility of morphine-induced premature aging.[21]

REFERENCES

1. Van der Laan JW, de Groot G. Changes in locomotor activity patterns as a measure of spontaneous morphine withdrawal: No effect of clonidine. Drug Alcohol Depend 1988; 22:133-140.
2. Van der Laan JW, Land CJ, Loeber JG et al. Validation of spontaneous morphine withdrawal symptoms in rats. Arch Int Pharmacodyn Ther 1991; 311:42-45.
3. Gellert VF, Holtzman SG. Development and maintenance of morphine tolerance and dependence in the rat by scheduled access to morphine drinking solutions. J Pharmacol Exp Ther 1978; 205:536-546.
4. Auriacombe M, Tignol J, Le Moal M et al. Transcutaneous electrical stimulation with limoge current potentiates morphine analgesia and attenuates opiate abstinence syndrome. Biol Psychiatry 1990; 28:650-656.
5. Meltzer LT, Moreton JE, Khazan N. Electroencephalographic and behavioral tolerance and cross-tolerance to morphine and metha-

done in the rat. Toxicol Appl Pharmacol 1978; 45:837-844.

6. Weeks JR. Experimental morphine addiction: Method for automatic intravenous injections in unrestrained rats. Science 1962; 138: 143-144.

7. Gold LH, Stinus L, Inturrisi CE et al. Prolonged tolerance, dependence and abstinence following subcutaneous morphine pellet implantation in the rat. Eur J Pharmacol 1994; 253:45-51.

8. Yoburn BC, Chen T, Huang T et al. Pharmacokinetic and pharmacodynamics of subcutaneous morphine pellets in the rat. J Pharmacol Exp Ther 1985; 235:282-286.

9. Bläsig J, Herz A, Reinhold K et al. Development of physical dependence on morphine with respect to time and dosage and quantification of the precipitated withdrawal syndrome in rats. Psychopharmacologia 1973; 33:19-38.

10. Cerletti C, Keinath SH, Reidenberg MM et al. Chronic morphine administration: Plasma levels and withdrawal syndrome in rats. Pharmacol Biochem Behav 1976; 4:323-327.

11. Maldonado R, Feger J, Fournié-Zaluski MC et al. Differences in physical dependence induced by selective mu or delta opioid agonists and by endogenous enkephalins protected by peptidase inhibitors. Brain Res 1990; 520:247-254.

12. Wei E, Loh HH, Way EL. Quantitative aspects of precipitated abstinence in morphine-dependent rats. J Pharmacol Exp Ther 1973; 184:398-403.

13. Schulteis G, Markou A, Gold L et al. Relative sensitivity to naloxone of multiple indices of opiate withdrawal: A quantitative dose-response analysis. J Pharmacol Exp Ther 1994; 271:1391-1398.

14. Stinus L, Allard M, Gold L et al. Changes in CNS neuropeptide FF-like material, pain sensitivity and opiate dependence following chronic morphine treatment. Peptides 1995; 16:1235-1241.

15. Espejo EF, Cador M, Stinus L. Ethopharmacological analysis of naloxone-precipitated morphine withdrawal syndrome in rats: A newly developed "etho-score". Psychopharmacology 1995; 122: 122-130.

16. Jaffe JH. Drug addiction and drug abuse. In: Gilman AG, Goodman LS, Rall TW, eds. Goodman and Gilman's The Pharmacological Basis of Therapeutics. 7th ed. New York: MacMillan Publishing Co., 1990:522-573.

17. Henningfield JE, Johnson RE, Jasinski DR. Clinical procedures for the assessment of abuse potential. In: Bozarth MA, ed. Methods of Assessing the Reinforcing Properties of Abused Drugs. New York: Springer-Verlag, 1987:573-590.

18. Jasinski DR, Johnson RE, Kocher TR. Clonidine in morphine withdrawal: Differential effects of signs and symptoms. Arch Gen Psy-

chiatry 1985; 42:1063-1066.

19. Stinus L. Neurobiological aspects of opiate dependence. In: Stefanis C, Hippius H, eds. Psychiatry in Progress: Research in Addiction, Vol. 2. Seattle: Hogrefe and Huber Publishing, 1995:1-21.

20. Martin WR, Wikler A, Eades CG et al. Tolerance to and physical dependence on morphine in rats. Psychopharmacologia 1963; 4:247-260.

21. Sala M, Braida D, Leone MP et al. Chronic morphine affects working memory during treatment and withdrawal in rats: Possible residual long-term impairment. Behav Pharmacol 1994; 5:570-580.

22. Babbini M, Gaiardi M, Bartoletti M. Persistence of chronic morphine effects upon activity in rats 8 months after ceasing the treatment. Neuropharmacology 1975; 14:611-614.

23. Brady L, Holtzman SG. Locomotor activity in morphine-dependent and post-dependent rats. Pharmacol Biochem Behav 1981; 14:361-370.

24. Koob GF, Wall TL, Bloom FE. Nucleus accumbens as a substrate for the aversive stimulus effects of opiate withdrawal. Psychopharmacology (Berlin) 1989; 98:530-534.

25. Markou A, Koob GF. Post-cocaine anhedonia. An animal model of cocaine withdrawal. Neuropharmacology 1991; 4:17-26.

26. Negus SS, Pasternak GW, Koob GF et al. Antagonist effect of β-funaltrexamine and naloxonazine on alfentanil-induced antinociception and muscle rigidity in the rat. J Pharmacol Exp Ther 1993; 264:739-745.

27. Kornetsky C, Esposito RU. Euphorigenic drugs: Effects on reward pathways of the brain. Fed Proc 1979; 38:2473-2476.

28. Perry W, Esposito RU, Kornetsky C. Effects of chronic naloxone treatment on brain stimulation reward. Pharmacol Biochem Behav 1981; 14:247-249.

29. Oswald I, Evans JI, Lewis SA. Addictive drugs cause suppression of paradoxical sleep with withdrawal rebound. In: Steinberg H, ed. Scientific Basis of Drug Dependence. London: J and A Churchill, 1969:243-257.

30. Khazan N. EEG correlates of morphine dependence and withdrawal in the rat. In: Singh JM, Miller LH, Al H, eds. Experimental Pharmacology. New York: Futura Publishing House, 1972:159-172.

31. Colasanti B, Kirchman A, Khazan N. Changes in the electroencephalogram and REM sleep time during morphine abstinence in pellet-implanted rats. Res Commun Chem Pathol Pharmacol 1975; 12:163-172.

32. Khazan N, Colasanti B. EEG correlates of morphine challenge in post-addict rats. Psychopharmacologia 1971; 22:56-63.

33. O'Brien C. Experimental analysis of conditioning factors in hu-

man narcotic addiction. Pharmacol Rev 1975; 27:533-543.

34. O'Brien C, Childress A, McLellan A et al. Learning factors in substance abuse, Ray BA (ed). NIDA Res Monogr 1988; 84:44-61.

35. Higgins GA, Nguyen P, Joharchi N et al. Effects of 5-HT3 receptor antagonists on behavioral measures of naloxone-precipitated opioid withdrawal. Psychopharmacology 1991; 105:322-328.

36. Mucha RF. Is the motivational effect of opiate withdrawal reflected by common somatic indices of precipitated withdrawal? Brain Res 1987; 418:214-220.

37. Stinus L, Le Moal M, Koob GF. The nucleus accumbens and amygdala as possible substrates for the aversive stimulus effects of opiate withdrawal. Neuroscience 1990; 37:767-773.

38. Hand TH, Koob GF, Stinus L et al. Aversive properties of opiate receptor blockade are centrally mediated and are potentiated by previous exposure to opiates. Brain Res 1988; 474:364-368.

39. Hand TH, Stinus L, Le Moal M. Differential mechanisms in the acquisition and expression of heroin-induced place preference. Psychopharmacology 1989; 98:61-67.

40. Baldwin HA, Koob GF. Rapid induction of conditioned opiate withdrawal. Neuropsychopharmacology 1993; 8:15-21.

41. Heishman SJ, Stitzer ML, Bigelow GE et al. Acute opioid physical dependence in humans: Effect of varying the morphine-naloxone interval. J Pharmacol Exp Ther 1989; 250:485-491.

42. Azorlosa JL, Stitzer ML, Greenwald MK. Opioid physical dependence development: Effects of single versus repeated morphine pretreatments and of subjects' opioid exposure history. Psychopharmacology 1994; 114:71-80.

43. Kim DH, Fields HL, Barbaro NM. Morphine analgesia and acute physical dependence: Rapid onset of two opposing dose-related processes. Brain Res 1990; 516:37-40.

44. Hendrie CA. Naloxone-sensitive hyperalgesia follows analgesia induced by morphine and environmental stimulation. Pharmacol Biochem Behav 1989; 32:961-966.

45. Kanof PD, Aronson MJ, Ness R et al. Levels of opioid physical dependence in heroin addicts. Drug Alcohol Depend 1991; 27:253-262.

46. Babbini M, Davis WM. Time-dose relationship for locomotor activity effects of morphine after acute or repeated treatment. Br J Pharmacol 1972; 46:213-224.

47. Young GA, Khazan N. Differential protracted effects of morphine and ethylketocylazocine challenges on EEG and behavior in the rat. Eur J Pharmacol 1986; 125:265-271.

48. Gianutsos G, Hynes MD, Drawbauch RB et al. Morphine withdrawal aggression during protracted abstinence: Role of latent

dopaminergic supersensitivity. Pharmacologist 1973; 15:348.

49. Gianutsos G, Hynes MD, Puri SK et al. Effect of apomorphine and nigrostriatal lesions on aggression and striatal dopamine turnover during morphine withdrawal: Evidence for dopaminergic supersentivitiy in protracted abstinence. Psychopharmacologia 1974; 34:37-44.

50. Spain JW, Newsom GC. Chronic opioids impair acquisition of both radial maze and Y-maze choice escape. Psychopharmacology 1991; 105:101-106.

================= CHAPTER 3 =================

NEUROPHYSIOLOGY
OF OPIATE DEPENDENCE

REGIONAL CEREBRAL GLUCOSE UTILIZATION DURING OPIATE DEPENDENCE

The physiological activity of neurons requires energy derived from the metabolism of glucose. The mapping and quantification of regional glucose utilization rates by the 2-deoxy-D-[1-^{14}C] glucose is a method that provides an index of regional functional activity in the central nervous system.[1] This method has been used to investigate the functional cerebral anatomy of both spontaneous and naloxone-precipitated morphine withdrawal. A selective and highly reproducible enhancement on rates of glucose utilization was found during morphine withdrawal.[2-4] The regional distribution of this elevated metabolic activity was similar during spontaneous and naloxone-precipitated withdrawal, but a smaller magnitude of changes overall was observed in spontaneous withdrawal that could reflect its reduced behavioral intensity compared to precipitated withdrawal.[3] The hypermetabolism was primarily produced in thalamic and limbic areas, particularly the central nucleus of amygdala. Several hypothalamic nuclei, including the posterior nucleus, the paraventricular nucleus and the lateral area, showed increased metabolic activity. Other midbrain regions, such as locus coeruleus, ventral tegmental area, dorsal parabrachial nucleus, superior colliculus, dorsal tegmental nucleus and median raphe, also increased their glucose utilization rates. Cortical areas (except visual and olfactory cortices) and hindbrain (excluding cerebellar vermis) were almost unaffected.[4] Low doses of naloxone (0.5 µg/kg) insufficient to produce severe behavioral signs of withdrawal in

dependent rats were able to increase rates of glucose utilization in
the thalamic nuclei and certain brain stem structures such as the
interpeduncular nucleus.[3] The enhancement in metabolic activity
during morphine abstinence was found in many noradrenergic
structures[4] in agreement with previous results obtained after local
administration of opiate antagonists[5] and c-fos mapping,[6] suggesting the involvement of the noradrenergic system in opiate dependence and withdrawal. In addition, during precipitated morphine
withdrawal, an increased glucose utilization was found in the superficial layers of the dorsal horn in the cervical and thoracic spinal cord. This hypermetabolism could be due to an increased input from small diameter primary afferent fibers, and it supports
the hypothesis that the enhanced neuronal activity in superficial
layers of the spinal cord participates in the manifestation of opioid
withdrawal.[7]

Acute and chronic morphine exposure has been reported to
induce effects opposite those of morphine withdrawal, i.e., a decrease in the rate of glucose utilization in some selective brain structures. Thus, acute morphine exposure produces metabolic decreases
in several thalamic nuclei,[8] whereas chronic treatment diminishes
glucose utilization in cortical regions.[4] Early studies, however, reported a small increase in metabolism in chronically morphine-
treated rats and a return toward control during withdrawal in some
brain regions such as dorsal hippocampus, entorhinal cortex and
subiculum.[2] The discrepancies could be due to the appearance of
opioid withdrawal in chronically morphine-treated animals since
rates of glucose utilization were measured some hours after the
removal of morphine pellets in this study.[2]

The increased brain rates of glucose utilization during naloxone-
precipitated morphine withdrawal have been reported to be reduced
by compounds that are able to attenuate the behavioral expression
of morphine abstinence, such as the α_2-agonist clonidine.[9] This
effect is a widespread phenomenon that affects brain regions containing high densities of α_2-receptors, mainly hypothalamic nuclei
and limbic areas, and other structures with very low densities of
these receptors. However, the distribution of the metabolic responses to specific drugs is usually not related simply to the presence of relevant receptors but also reflects the influence of affer-

ents to the areas evaluated.[10] Consequently, other regions different from locus coeruleus could participate in the beneficial action of clonidine on the opioid abstinence syndrome.

The effects produced on brain metabolism during the morphine withdrawal syndrome precipitated by the local administration of an opiate antagonist into specific brain structures have also been recently investigated. The local administration of the hydrophilic antagonist methylnaloxonium into the locus coeruleus in morphine-dependent rats induced large metabolic increases in thalamus, limbic areas, hypothalamus, mammillary nucleus, midbrain areas and cerebellar vermis. The regional distribution of the elevated metabolic activity after the local administration into this noradrenergic structure was very similar to that observed after the systemic injection of opiate antagonists. However, no changes in glucose utilization in any of the regions assayed were found when the opiate antagonist was injected into the amygdala. These results suggest that many metabolic changes throughout the brain produced by opioid withdrawal may be secondary to events that begin in the locus coeruleus.[11]

ROLE OF THE INTRACELLULAR MESSENGER PATHWAYS ON THE ADAPTIVE CHANGES INDUCED BY CHRONIC OPIATE EXPOSURE

Many neurotransmitters in the brain, including opioid peptides and opiate drugs, bind to receptor proteins that do not contain ion channels within their structures. Instead, these receptors produce their physiological effects via interacting with G-proteins which are referred to as G-protein-coupled receptors, e.g., they bind guanine nucleotides. Upon binding of neurotransmitter or drug to the receptor, the receptor becomes associated with the G-protein which allows the G-protein subunits to interact with many other cellular proteins to produce various physiological effects. One target of the G-protein subunits is a direct action on ion channels. Opioid peptides can increase the activity of certain K^+ channels and decrease the activity of certain Ca^{2+} channels through these G-protein mechanisms.[12] Both of these actions on channels are considered inhibitory actions because more K^+ flows out of the cell and less Ca^{2+} flows into the cell, and these effects may mediate the relatively rapid effects of opiates on the electrical properties of their target neurons.

Another action of G-protein-coupled receptors is to influence other neural processes through complex pathways of intracellular messengers. The first step in these pathways are "second messengers" which include cAMP, cGMP, Ca^{2+}, nitric oxide, prostaglandins and phosphatidylinositol. G-protein-coupled receptors control the activity of these second messengers by regulating the activity of enzymes that catalyze the synthesis and degradation of second messengers. Opioid peptides and opiates decrease cAMP levels by acting through an inhibitory G-protein (Gi), which binds to and inhibits adenylyl cyclase, the enzyme that catalyzes the synthesis of cAMP.[12]

The cellular site of opiate actions had long been hypothesized to involve actions on second messenger systems that include modification of cyclic AMP, and that these changes were altered as part of an adaptation to the chronic administration of the drug. According to this hypothesis, inhibition by an opiate of a process in a second messenger system could lead to tolerance and dependence through a compensating "hypertrophy" in this same system.[13,14] The affinity of opiates for the opiate receptor is correlated with their ability to acutely inhibit adenylate cyclase,[15] and neuroblastoma x glioma hybrid cells (NG 108-15 cells), cultured in the presence of an opiate, develop tolerance and dependence as reflected in an increased production of cyclic AMP under certain situations.[15,16]

Several other early results supported the hypothesis of an activation of cyclic AMP in the neurons of dependent animals. Opiate withdrawal increases brain cyclic AMP levels.[17] Injection of cyclic AMP intracerebroventricularly in dependent rats increased naloxone-induced withdrawal jumping.[18] Protein kinase activity was increased in the brain during opiate withdrawal.[19] Finally, a quasi-withdrawal syndrome could be induced in opiate-naive rats by treatment with phosphodiesterase inhibitors.[20]

Subsequent studies have extended these early whole brain studies to specific structures in the central nervous system (CNS) that have been implicated in opiate withdrawal (see chapter 5). In a whole series of elegant studies, Nestler and coworkers have demonstrated that, in the noradrenergic nucleus of the locus coeruleus (LC), acute morphine treatment decreases the activity of the second messenger system, e.g., cyclic AMP system, at all levels of biochemical transduction of the physiological response, and chronic morphine treatment upregulates the cyclic AMP system at every major step between receptor and response,[12,21,22] including protein kinase[22] and G-proteins[21] (Fig. 3.1).

The next step in these intracellular pathways, the regulation by second messengers of protein phosphorylation, provides a further means of explaining the neuroadaptation associated with opiate dependence. Many types of proteins are regulated by phosphorylation, including phosphorylation of cytoskeletal proteins which affects the size and shape of neurons, and phosphorylation of nuclear proteins which affects their ability to regulate gene expression. These changes presumably include those that may trigger the longer-term effects of the drugs which eventually lead to tolerance, dependence, withdrawal and addiction.

A model system for these neuroadaptive changes is the nucleus a locus coeruleus, the major noradrenergic nucleus in the brain, which plays an important role in physical dependence to opiates (see chapter 5). Activation of the locus coeruleus has been shown to mediate many of the signs and symptoms of opiate withdrawal in animals.[23-26]

Withdrawal activation of the locus coeruleus is likely due to a combination of factors within and outside of the locus coeruleus system that influence its excitability. The outside factors include activation of the major glutamatergic input to the locus coeruleus which projects from a brain stem area, the paragigantocellularis.[27,28] Mechanisms within the locus coeruleus system itself may involve upregulation of the cAMP pathway described above.[12,15,29] Acutely, opiates inhibit the cAMP pathway in the LC by inhibiting adenylyl cyclase, a molecular site of action for opiate neuroadaptation described above. In contrast, chronic exposure to opiates increases the amount of adenylyl cyclase and cAMP-dependent protein kinase expressed in these neurons. This upregulated cAMP pathway has been shown to contribute to the increase in the electrical excitability of locus coeruleus neurons associated with withdrawal.[12]

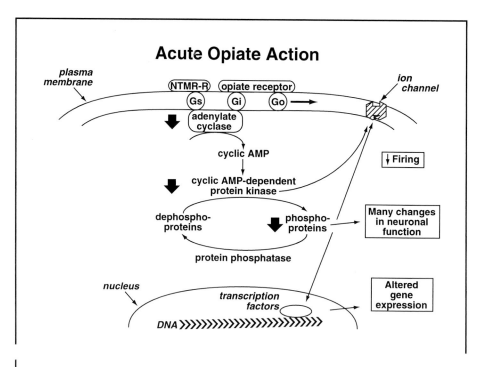

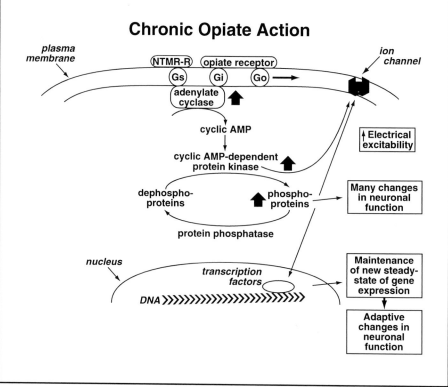

Fig. 3.1 (opposite). Schematic illustration of the hypothetical mechanisms of acute and chronic opiate action in brain sites involved in opiate dependence such as the locus coeruleus and nucleus accumbens. Top, Opiates acutely inhibit neurons via coupling with a pertussis toxin-inhibitable G-protein (perhaps G_O), and by decreasing the conductance of a nonspecific cation channel (hatched) via coupling with G_i (the inhibitory G-protein) and the consequent inhibition of the cAMP pathway (large downward arrows) and reduced phosphorylation of the channel or a closely associated protein. Inhibition of the cAMP pathway via decreased phosphorylation of numerous other proteins would affect many processes in the neuron; in addition to reducing firing rates, for example, it would initiate alterations in gene expression via regulation of transcription factors. Bottom, Chronic administration of opiates leads to a compensatory upregulation of the cAMP pathway (large upward arrows) which contributes to opiate dependence in the neurons by increasing their intrinsic excitability via increased activation of the nonspecific cation channel. In addition, upregulation of the cAMP pathway presumably would be associated with persistent changes in transcription factors that maintain the chronic morphine-treated state. Modified from Nestler.[12]

Much less is known about the role of intracellular messenger systems in the motivational aspects of dependence, although there is some evidence to suggest that similar mechanisms may be involved. Opiates do upregulate the cAMP pathway in the nucleus accumbens after chronic administration.[12,30,31] In addition, studies involving direct administration of activators or inhibitors of the cAMP pathway into the nucleus accumbens are consistent with the interpretation that upregulation of the cAMP pathway in this brain region may contribute to an aversive state during drug withdrawal.[31]

Finally, the activation of second messenger and protein phosphorylation pathways may lead to the phosphorylation of certain transcription factors which then stimulate transcriptional activity and, ultimately, changes in early gene expression. One example of such a stimulation of transcription is the activation of cAMP response element binding (CREB) protein, which is phosphorylated and activated by cAMP- and Ca^{2+}-dependent protein kinases. Activation of CREB and related proteins could then stimulate new synthesis of additional transcription factors. For example, c-fos and many related proteins, which are normally present at very low levels in the brain, are activated dramatically in response to cAMP, Ca^{2+} and other second messenger signals and can be induced within minutes of an acute stimulus (see below). The genes coding for c-fos and related proteins are termed "immediate-early genes"[32] and are clearly activated during opiate withdrawal (see below).

STUDIES ON C-FOS EXPRESSION
DURING OPIATE DEPENDENCE

The c-fos proto-oncogene product, Fos, is a nuclear protein which, in complex with other nuclear proteins such as Jun, binds to DNA and appears to regulate the transcription of specific cellular genes. In the CNS, the expression of c-fos mRNA and protein is stimulated rapidly in response to increases in neuronal activity, and thus these nuclear proteins are termed "immediate-early genes." For this reason opiate regulation of the nuclear proto-oncogene c-fos has been studied in CNS by immunoblotting, northern blotting and in situ hybridization procedures in order to detect neuronal activations triggered by naloxone-precipitated opiate withdrawal in rats. This experimental approach is complementary to 2-deoxy-glucose autoradiographic procedures, but unlike 2-deoxy-glucose, which reflects glucose metabolism primarily in nerve terminals, c-fos reflects physiological activity in cell bodies. Levels of c-fos expression are depressed by chronic morphine treatment.

In contrast, naloxone-precipitated opiate withdrawal, which increases LC firing rate 4-fold, leads to a +170% increase in levels of mRNA and protein c-fos in LC 1-2 hours after the initiation of withdrawal. Similar regulation of c-fos expression during opiate withdrawal was found in neostriatum, cerebral cortex and in limbic structures such as amygdaloid complex, ventral tegmental area and nucleus accumbens. Negative results were obtained in other brain regions studied including the hippocampus, dorsal raphe, periaqueductal gray and paragigantocellularis nucleus which gives rise to the enkephalinergic innervation of LC.[6] In LC and amygdala, induction of c-fos during opiate withdrawal was associated with a parallel induction of c-jun, another nuclear proto-oncogene. While a dramatic increase in mRNA levels for c-fos was observed in LC during opiate withdrawal, mRNA levels for tyrosine hydroxylase, the rate-limiting enzyme in catecholamine synthesis, and for precursors to galanin and neuropeptide Y, peptides that coexist with norepinephrine in LC neurons, were not altered by naloxone-precipitated withdrawal in morphine-dependent rats.[33]

Using c-fos-like immunoreactivity (CFIR), other authors confirmed the neuronal activation induced by precipitated opiate withdrawal in LC and ventral tegmental area, as evidenced by the in-

Table 3.1. Regulation of c-fos expression during opiate withdrawal in rat brain

Brain Region	Levels of c-fos mRNA [% Control ± SEM (n)]
Locus coeruleus	272 ± 36 (4)*
Amygdala	180 ± 12 (4)*
Ventral tegmentum	259 ± 26 (4)*
Nucleus accumbens	234 ± 20 (4)*
Neostriatum	217 ± 10 (4)*
Cerebral cortex	238 ± 20 (6)*
Frontal cortex	193 ± 9 (4)*
Pons	95 ± 10 (4)
Paragigantocellularis	103 ± 7 (5)
Hippocampus	109 ± 11 (3)
Dorsal raphe	109 ± 17 (2)
Periacqueductal gray	105 ± 12 (3)

*$p < 0.05$ by χ^2-test
Levels of c-fos mRNA in various regions of the rat brain were quantified with Northern blotting. Animals were made dependent on opiates by subcutaneous implantation of morphine pellets (75 mg, NIDA). Opiate withdrawal was precipitated by a single subcutaneous injection of naltrexone (100 mg/kg). Animals were killed 1 hour after the naltrexone injection. Reproduced with permission from Hayward MD et al, Brain Res 1990; 525:256-266.

crease of the number of CFIR-positive neurons in these regions (Table 3.1). Moreover, they found a significant increase in the number of CFIR-containing neurons within the caudal ventrolateral portion of periaqueductal gray.[34] These regions showing c-fos immunoreactivity during opiate withdrawal are those involved in the rewarding effects of opiates and in integration of autonomic and somatic components of defensive and escape behaviors which are characteristic signs of opiate withdrawal. Further experiments are needed to characterize these neuronal populations and to know if their activation is the neurobiological substrate or the consequence of opiate withdrawal.

REFERENCES

1. Sokoloff L, Reivich M, Kennedy C et al. The [14C] deoxyglucose method for measurement of local cerebral glucose utilization: Theory, procedure and normal values in the conscious and anesthetized albino rat. J Neurochem 1977; 28:897-916.

2. Wooten GF, DiStefano P, Collins RC. Regional cerebral glucose utilization during morphine withdrawal in the rat. Proc Natl Acad Sci USA 1982; 79:3360-3364.

3. Geary WA II, Wooten GF. Similar functional anatomy of spontaneous and precipitated morphine withdrawal. Brain Res 1985; 334:183-186.

4. Kimes AS, London ED. Glucose utilization in the rat brain during chronic morphine treatment and naloxone-precipitated morphine withdrawal. J Pharmacol Exp Ther 1989; 248:538-545.

5. Maldonado R, Stinus L, Gold LH et al. Role of different brain structures in the expression of the physical morphine withdrawal syndrome. J Pharmacol Exp Ther 1992; 261:669-677.

6. Hayward MD, Duman RS, Nestler EJ. Induction of the c-fos proto-oncogene during opiate withdrawal in the locus coeruleus and other regions of rat brain. Brain Res 1990; 525:256-266.

7. Bell JA, Kimes AS, London ED. Increased glucose utilization in superficial layers of the rat spinal dorsal horn during precipitated morphine withdrawal. Eur J Pharmacol 1988; 150:171-174.

8. Fanelli RJ, Szikszay M, Jasinski DR et al. Differential effects of mu and kappa opioid analgesics on cerebral glucose utilization in the rat. Brain Res 1987; 422:257-266.

9. Kimes AS, Bell JA, London ED. Clonidine attenuates increased brain glucose metabolism during naloxone-precipitated morphine withdrawal. Neuroscience 1990; 34:633-644.

10. McCulloch J. Mapping functional alterations in the CNS with [^{14}C] deoxyglucose. In: Iversen LL, Iversen SD, Snyder SH, eds. Handbook of Psychopharmacology, Vol. 15. New York: Plenum Press, 1982:321-410.

11. Kimes AS, Maldonado R, Koob GF et al. Cerebral glucose metabolism during opioid withdrawal following methylnaloxonium injection into the locus coeruleus. Synapse 1996; (in press).

12. Nestler EJ. Molecular mechanisms of drug addiction. J Neurosci 1992; 12:2439-2450.

13. Collier HOJ, Roy AC. Morphine-like drugs inhibit the stimulation by E prostaglandins of cyclic AMP formation by rat brain homogenate. Nature 1974; 248:24-27.

14. Collier HOJ. Cellular site of opiate dependence. Nature 1980; 283:625-630.

15. Sharma SK, Klee WA, Nirenberg M. Dual regulation of adenylate cyclase accounts for narcotic dependence and tolerance. Proc Natl Acad Sci USA 1975; 72:3092-3096.

16. Traber J, Gullis R, Hamprecht B. Influence of opiates on the levels of adenosine 3'5'-cyclic monophosphate in neuroblastoma x glioma hybrid cells. Life Sci 1975; 16:1863-1868.

17. Collier HOJ, Francis DL, McDonald-Gibson WJ et al. Prostaglandins, cyclic AMP and the mechanism of opiate dependence. Life Sci 1975; 17:85-90.

18. Collier HOJ, Francis DL. Morphine abstinence is associated with increased brain cyclic AMP. Nature 1975; 255:159-162.

19. Clark AG, Jovic R, Ornellas MR et al. Brain microsomal protein kinase in the chronically morphinized rat. Biochem Pharmacol 1972; 21:1989-1990.

20. Francis DL, Roy AC, Collier HOJ. Morphine abstinence and quasi-abstinence effects after phosphodiesterase inhibitors and naloxone. Life Sci 1975; 16:1901-1906.

21. Nestler EJ, Erdos JJ, Terwilliger R et al. Regulation of G-proteins by chronic morphine in the rat locus coeruleus. Brain Res 1989; 476:230-239.

22. Nestler EJ, Tallman JF. Chronic morphine treatment increases cyclic AMP-dependent protein kinase activity in the rat locus coeruleus. Mol Pharmacol 1988; 33:127-132.

23. Aghajanian GK. Tolerance of locus coeruleus neurons to morphine and suppression of withdrawal response by clonidine. Nature 1978; 276:186-188.

24. Koob GF, Maldonado R, Stinus L. Neural substrates of opiate withdrawal. Trends Neurosci 1992; 15:186-191.

25. Rasmussen K, Beitner-Johnson DB, Krystal JH et al. Opiate withdrawal and rat locus coeruleus: Behavioral, electrophysiological, and biochemical correlates. J Neurosci 1990; 10:2308-2317.

26. Taylor JR, Elsworth JD, Garcia EJ et al. Clonidine infusions into the locus coeruleus attenuate behavioral and neurochemical changes associated with naloxone-precipitated withdrawal. Psychopharmacology 1988; 96:121-131.

27. Rasmussen K, Aghajanian GK. Withdrawal-induced activation of locus coeruleus neurons in opiate-dependent rats: Attenuation by lesion of the nucleus paragigantocellularis. Brain Res 1989; 505:346-350.

28. Akaoka H, Aston-Jones G. Opiate withdrawal-induced hyperactivity of locus coeruleus neurons is substantially mediated by augmented excitatory acid input. J Neurosci 1991; 11:3830-3839.

29. Nestler EJ, Hope BT, Widnell KL. Drug addiction: A model for the molecular basis of neural plasticity. Neuron 1993; 11:995-1006.

30. Terwilliger R, Beitner-Johnson D, Sevarino KA et al. A general role for adaptations in G-proteins and cyclic AMP system in mediating the chronic actions of morphine and cocaine on neuronal function. Brain Res 1991; 548:100-110.

31. Self DW, Nestler EJ. Molecular mechanisms of drug reinforcement and craving. Annu Rev Neurosci 1995; 18:463-495.

32. Morgan JI, Curran T. Stimulus-transcription coupling in the nervous system: Involvement of the inducible proto-oncogenes fos and jun. Annu Rev Neurosci 1991; 14:421-451.

33. Holmes PV, Bartolomeis A, Koprivica V et al. Lack of effect of chronic morphine treatment and naloxone-precipitated withdrawal on tyrosine hydroxylase, galanin and neuropeptide Y mRNA levels in rat locus coeruleus. Synapse 1995; 19:197-205.

34. Chieng B, Keay KA, Christie MDJ. Increased fos-like immunoreactivity in the periaqueductal gray of anaesthetized rats during opiate withdrawal. Neurosci Lett 1995; 183:79-82.

CHAPTER 4

NEUROCHEMISTRY
OF OPIATE DEPENDENCE

The neurochemical mechanisms implicated in the development of opiate dependence and the expression of withdrawal syndrome include processes of homologous regulation affecting the endogenous opioid system and heterologous regulation that affects other neurotransmitter systems.[1] Numerous nonopioid systems have been proposed to participate in this heterologous regulation. Thus, changes in several classical neurotransmitters and neuropeptides have been reported during chronic opiate administration and at the moment of spontaneous or naloxone-precipitated morphine abstinence. This chapter focuses on the changes observed in the noradrenergic and dopaminergic systems in order to explain the role of these heterologous regulation processes in the expression of the different components of opioid withdrawal. Their involvement is supported by several lines of evidence based on the biochemical changes reported in these neurotransmitters during opiate dependence and withdrawal, and on the pharmacological responses induced on opiate withdrawal by the administration of compounds able to modify the activity of these systems.

CHANGES ON NORADRENALINE CONTENT
AND RELEASE DURING OPIATE DEPENDENCE

Multiple studies have shown the involvement of the central noradrenergic system in the adaptive changes occurring during the development of opiate dependence. The first evidence was reported by studies on noradrenaline (NA) and metabolite levels in brain, plasma and urine during chronic morphine treatment and after precipitation of withdrawal syndrome, and suggested the presence of a noradrenergic hyperactivity during opiate withdrawal. However, the significance of these early findings is limited since the measurement of the total content in the brain and the plasma or urinary level of catecholamines are not good indicators of central noradrenergic activity. Another biochemical technique used was the measurement of NA release from in vitro brain slice preparations. The results obtained by using this method also suggest an increase in noradrenergic activity during opiate abstinence. The recent development of in vivo microdialysis techniques in freely moving rats allows the measurement of the extracellular concentrations of neurotransmitters in discrete areas of the central nervous system, which is a direct reflection of the synaptic release of these transmitters. The use of this technique has clarified the significance of the previous findings reported on NA content and confirmed the results obtained using in vitro brain slice preparations.

NORADRENALINE AND METABOLITE LEVELS

Early studies reported marked alterations in the catecholamine content of brain, adrenals and urine during chronic morphine treatment and after withdrawal. The results obtained in these studies were contradictory in some cases, probably as a consequence of the different animal species and protocols used. However, they provided the first evidence of a hyperactivity of the noradrenergic system during opiate withdrawal. Acute morphine administration was associated with a decrease of NA levels in the brain and adrenalin in the adrenal glands, together with an increased urinary output of catecholamines, suggesting a releasing effect of morphine under acute conditions.[2-5] It was observed that during chronic morphine treatment, catecholamines in brain and adrenals tended to return to control levels, and the urinary excretion stabilized at a slightly elevated rate which was maintained as long as morphine was given.[3-7] These findings suggested that the adaptation to long-term chronic exposure of morphine was associated with a reduced liberation of catecholamines and a stimulated resynthesis compared to the acute conditions. Spontaneous and precipitated morphine withdrawal was associated with a reduction of NA in the brain, of adrenaline in the adrenal glands, and an increased urinary output of catecholamines.[3-5,7,8] The decrease in brain NA was directly related to the degree of morphine withdrawal, and the maximal urinary output of catecholamines was reached at the same time as the maximal intensity of abstinence.[3,4] These findings suggested that a rapid release of catecholamines in brain and adrenals occurs during withdrawal, which was related to the expression of some excitatory signs of abstinence.

Noradrenaline utilization (α-methylparatyrosine-induced disappearance) has also been investigated during opiate treatment and withdrawal. Acute morphine decreased NA utilization in several brain structures, and these changes disappeared during chronic treatment. No modification or variable changes were reported during morphine withdrawal depending on the brain area evaluated.[9] Other studies have investigated the brain content of the 3-methoxy-4-hydroxy-phenethyleneglycol (MHPG), the principal metabolite of brain NA. An enhancement in the brain content of MHPG was found in several brain regions innervated by the locus coeruleus during morphine abstinence[10] and was correlated with the severity of withdrawal behavior.[11] This increase in the NA metabolite levels in several brain structures was confirmed by other authors.[12-14] Clinical studies have also provided the same evidence. Thus, a relationship between increased MHPG plasma levels and the behavioral expression of naltrexone-precipitated withdrawal has been found in methadone-dependent humans.[15] Therefore, these results are in agreement with earlier studies that also reported an increased noradrenergic activity during opiate withdrawal.

STUDIES ON IN VITRO RELEASE

The acute administration of morphine depressed the release of NA on slice preparations from several brain structures such as cortex,[16,17] thalamus,[18,19] amygdala,[20] hippocampus and cerebellum.[17] This effect selectively involved an activation of μ-opioid receptors since it was observed after the administration of μ-, but not δ- or κ-, selective opioid agonists.[17,21,22] Chronic opioid administration resulted in a tolerance to morphine response expressed by a decrease in the ability of the opioid agonist to inhibit the release of

NA.[23] During opiate withdrawal, a rebound effect was reported on NA release. Thus, a spontaneous withdrawal was observed in cortical slices from morphine-dependent rats, as revealed by an increase in NA release when washing the slices, supporting the hypothesis of a noradrenergic hyperactivity during opiate abstinence.[16] A similar enhancement of NA release was reported by the addition of naloxone to brain slice preparations from morphine-dependent rats.[18,24] This increase seems to be due to adaptive changes on neuronal systems linked to μ-opioid receptors, rather than to the μ-opioid receptor itself whose sensitivity remains unchanged.[25] Consequently, the basic release mechanism responsible for the acute effects induced by opiates seems to be adapted to the continuous inhibition of release during chronic treatment with opiates. As a consequence of this adaptation, an increased release of NA occurs during opiate withdrawal.

IN VIVO MICRODIALYSIS STUDIES

Microdialysis studies have shown that acute morphine administration decreases the extraneuronal level of NA in the prefrontal cortex. Tolerance developed to this inhibitory effect during chronic morphine treatment, and morphine had no effect on NA output in dependent animals. The extraneuronal NA concentration was immediately enhanced after naloxone-precipitated morphine withdrawal syndrome, reaching maximal levels within 30 minutes after naloxone and remaining elevated for a period of 90 minutes. The symptomatology of withdrawal paralleled these changes in NA cortical output,[26] which is compatible with the previous hypothesis that some of the behavioral signs of abstinence may be mediated by an increased activity of the NA system.[3,4,27] An increase in NA output, without changes in serotonin or dopamine (DA) release, was also observed in the hippocampus after naloxone-precipitated abstinence.[28,29] In this case, the response was quantitatively stronger than that reported in cortical regions, and NA output remained increased 120 minutes after naloxone injection.[28] Therefore, these in vivo microdialysis studies confirmed the hypothesis postulated from previous biochemical results, suggesting the presence of a noradrenergic hyperactivity during the opiate withdrawal syndrome.

CHANGES IN DOPAMINE CONTENT AND RELEASE DURING OPIATE DEPENDENCE

Most of the early studies on dopamine (DA) and metabolite levels reported conflicting results during morphine treatment and withdrawal and did not provide any sound argument involving this neurotransmitter in opiate dependence. However, studies performed on DA release from in vitro brain slice preparations and in vivo microdialysis revealed that DA neurotransmission plays an important role in the acute and long-term effects of opiates, including the development of dependence. In general, the changes reported on DA release during opiate withdrawal are in opposition to those found on noradrenergic transmission, suggesting that a decreased dopaminergic activity could be related to several manifestations of the abstinence syndrome.

DOPAMINE AND METABOLITE LEVELS

Early studies reported no changes in the DA brain content after acute administration of morphine in rodents[30,31] and cats,[30,32] although a decrease was shown after acute morphine administration in mice.[33] Most of the studies also found that chronic administration of morphine was unable to modify brain DA levels in different animal species.[4,8,34,35] In contrast, an increase in urinary DA elimination was induced in rats by chronic morphine treatment.[6] During spontaneous opiate abstinence, an increase in brain DA content was observed 24 hours after the last morphine administration.[36] However, the results obtained during naloxone-precipitated morphine withdrawal syndrome were dependent on the animal species used. Thus, an increase in brain DA was observed in rodents[37] and monkeys,[8,34] whereas a decrease was reported in dogs.[4] Studies performed on DA synthesis and metabolism also reported conflicting results that were difficult to interpret. Acute morphine administration increased the brain levels of the DA metabolite homovanillic acid[32,38] and the incorporation of ^{14}C-tyrosine in dopaminergic neurons.[39,40] An increase in homovanillic acid content was also reported in the striatum during chronic morphine treatment.[11] Naloxone-precipitated withdrawal syndrome was shown to enhance the incorporation of ^{14}C-tyrosine on dopaminergic neurons[41] and the homovanillic acid content in the striatum.[11] Results obtained on DA turnover during morphine withdrawal were contradictory. Thus, some authors found an increase in DA utilization in substantia nigra,[42] striatum[42,43] and nucleus accumbens[9] during morphine withdrawal, whereas other studies found the opposite effect in some of these structures (substantia nigra,[9] striatum[44] and ventral tegmental area[9]) under similar conditions.

STUDIES ON IN VITRO RELEASE

Studies performed on in vitro release from brain slice preparations revealed that the effects of morphine treatment and withdrawal are different depending on the opioid receptor activated and the temporal pattern of opiate treatment, which could explain the conflicting results obtained when measuring DA and metabolite levels. Thus, acute opiate administration has been reported to decrease DA release from superfused slices of rat striatum,[21-23,45,46] nucleus accumbens, frontal cortex, olfactory tubercle,[47] thalamus[19] and hypothalamus.[48] However, this inhibitory effect is selectively mediated through κ opioid receptors, since the activation of μ or δ receptors did not affect DA release in brain slices.[21-23,45,46] In contrast to these results, some authors have reported an increased striatal DA release after δ opioid activation.[49,50] Acute opioids, through the activation of κ receptors, also inhibit DA release from cultured neurons of rat ventral mesencephalon, which is the brain region containing substantia nigra and ventral tegmental areas.[51] Chronic activation of opioid receptors in these cultured DA neurons induces neuronal supersensitivity, i.e., an increased DA release toward different stimuli.[52] After withdrawal of chronic morphine, the changes in the release of DA from superfused rat striatal slices were dependent on the temporal pattern of morphine administration. Thus, in the case of chronic morphine treatment (three daily injections of increasing doses of morphine), a decrease in DA release was observed 1 day and 3 weeks after withdrawal.[53,54] However, in the case of repeated morphine treatment (10 mg/kg once a day), a decrease in DA release was observed 1 day after withdrawal, whereas after 3 weeks the opposite effect (i.e., increased DA release) was found.[54]

In Vivo Microdialysis Studies

Microdialysis studies revealed that acute morphine administration increases DA output in the nucleus accumbens and striatum,[55,56] as it was previously reported by using a push-pull cannula procedure.[57] This effect appears to be mediated by the activation of μ- or δ-opioid receptors since κ activation results in an inhibition of DA release in these structures.[56] As previously reported, the findings on in vitro slice preparations suggest that the direct opioid control of DA release is mediated exclusively by the inhibitory action of κ receptors. Therefore, the stimulatory effect of morphine, through the activation of μ- or δ-opioid receptors, is likely to be a consequence of its inhibitory action on neurons which tonically inhibit dopaminergic neurons at the level of the nerve terminal and/or the cell bodies (for instance, by acting on GABA or glutamate, both abundantly present in dopaminergic regions).[58] Tolerance to the activational effects of morphine was observed in the nucleus accumbens during chronic morphine treatment.[59-61] After spontaneous abstinence, a profound depression of mesolimbic DA release occurs.[60,62] This change was observed to persist for a period of 7 days.[62] A similar decrease in mesolimbic DA release was reported after naloxone-precipitated withdrawal syndrome.[26,61,63]. The maximal effect was observed within 120 minutes after naloxone, but the DA output was still diminished 240 minutes after withdrawal precipitation.[26] On the basis of these changes, the DA decrease was interpreted as the neurochemical correlate of a "dysphoric" state rather than of the physical symptoms of abstinence.[26]

Changes in DA metabolism may also be related to the changes in the activity of the noradrenergic system during morphine abstinence. Thus, the prefrontal cortex possesses corticofugal excitatory neurons that innervate limbic structures and DA midbrain cell group regions,[64] and NA has an inhibitory action on some of these neurons.[65] Consequently, it is possible that withdrawal-induced increases in prefrontocortical NA may contribute to the depression of mesolimbic DA release.[26]

During opiate abstinence, tolerance to the DA-releasing effect of morphine on rat nucleus accumbens was observed during the

24 hours after the last administration. This tolerance was followed by a facilitated effect of morphine on DA release that persisted for several days to weeks after withdrawal from morphine.[62,66] This phenomenon has been related to the long-lasting behavioral sensitization observed after chronic opiate administration[67] and may be involved in compulsive drug-seeking behavior and relapse into drug abuse. This point will be addressed with more details in chapter 6 of this book.

EFFECTS OF PHARMACOLOGICAL COMPOUNDS ACTING ON THE AMINERGIC SYSTEM

COMPOUNDS ACTING ON α-ADRENOCEPTORS

Two main types of α-adrenoceptors have been designated: α_1, predominantly localized at the postsynaptic level, and α_2, present at postjunctional and prejunctional sites. Like the μ-opioid receptors, the α_2-adrenoceptors are coupled negatively to adenylyl cyclase, whereas α_1-adrenoceptors are mainly coupled to a different second messenger system, phospholipase C.[68] alpha2-adrenoceptors have been functionally related to several opioid-mediated responses and appear to be colocalized with opioid receptors in some areas such as the rat locus coeruleus, diencephalon and amygdala.[69]

The involvement of α_2-adrenoceptors in opiate dependence and withdrawal has been suggested to be largely due to the anti-withdrawal effects of α_2-adrenoceptor agonists. The use of the α_2-agonist clonidine for the detoxification of heroin addicts was initially proposed by Gold et al in 1978,[70] showing this compound to be remarkably effective at alleviating the withdrawal symptoms in humans. However, the general ability of clonidine to relieve opiate withdrawal in humans has been called into question. In later clinical studies, clonidine appeared to suppress mainly the symptoms related to hyperactivity of the sympathetic system but failed to suppress psychological symptoms such as anxiety and restlessness.[71]

Animal studies have actually demonstrated some conflicting effects of clonidine on morphine abstinence in rats, where clonidine reduced the intensity of most of the autonomic[72] and somatic symptoms of withdrawal, e.g., wet dog shakes and weight loss,[73-77] but intensified escape behavior,[73,75,76] and in some cases increased teeth-chattering[74,76] and hyperactivity.[73,77] It was suggested that the suppressive actions of clonidine are mediated by α_2-adrenoceptors and the potentiation effects by α_1-adrenoceptors.[78] However, several findings indicate that all the effects induced by clonidine on the withdrawal syndrome seem to be selectively mediated through the α_2-adrenoceptors: first, the doses of clonidine used in these studies are usually low and elicit very little effect on α_1-adrenoceptors; second, in comparing agonists of varying selectivity for α_1- and α_2-adrenoceptors, only selective α_2-agonists suppressed wet dog shakes and increased jumping, whereas selective α_1-agonists did neither;[79] and third, the co-administration of the α_1-antagonist prazosin or doxazosine did not modify the effects of clonidine, whereas the α_2-antagonist yohimbine blocked these effects.[79,80]

Several $_2$-receptor agonists (clonidine, guanfacine, azepexol, talipexole and UK 14,304) have been shown to produce different profiles of activity on opiate withdrawal signs, suggesting the existence of α_2-adrenoceptor subtypes with a different role in modulating the opiate withdrawal response, at which the agonists could show different preferences.[81] This is in agreement with molecular studies indicating the presence of three α_2-receptor subtypes which have tentatively been named α_{2A}-, α_{2B}- and α_{2C}-adrenoceptors.[68]

Alpha$_2$-adrenergic compounds are also able to modify the negative motivational aspects of withdrawal in animals. Thus, clonidine has been reported to attenuate the suppression of operant-conditioned behavior produced during opiate abstinence,[82,83] whereas yohimbine enhanced the suppression of this conditioned behavior.[82] Clonidine was also effective in reducing the aversive properties of opiate withdrawal, as assessed by the place conditioning procedure, and this effect was specific to the morphine-exposed state since clonidine did not induce place conditioning in nondependent animals.[77,84] The effects of clonidine were also investigated in associative processes related to opiate dependence, which may represent an experimental model of opiate craving and relapse. Thus, the re-exposure of opiate-dependent rats 5 days after abstinence to the environment previously associated with morphine elicited context-specific withdrawal symptoms. Clonidine administration reduced the context-specific withdrawal, suggesting that this compound could reduce the relapse in abstinent ex-addicts produced by returning to an environment previously associated with the opiate.[77]

Several biochemical and electrophysiological changes induced by opiate withdrawal have also been reported to be reversed by clonidine, such as the adrenal tyrosine-hydroxylase activity increase and NA depletion,[72] the rise of NA turnover in the locus coeruleus[12,13] and cortex,[85] the increase in locus coeruleus MHPG levels,[10,86] and the increased neuronal firing in the central amygdala[87] and locus coeruleus.[88] Clonidine also reduced the enhancement induced by morphine withdrawal on acetylcholine output in the nucleus accumbens,[89] NA output in hypothalamus[90] and hippocampus,[28,91] and glutamate and aspartate release in the locus coeruleus.[92] The increased brain rates of glucose utilization during naloxone-precipitated morphine withdrawal were also strongly attenuated by this α_2-agonist.[93]

In contrast to these findings, other biochemical and behavioral manifestations of opiate withdrawal were unaffected by the administration of clonidine. Clonidine was unable to reduce the enhanced plasma levels of β-endorphin and corticosterone during morphine withdrawal[90,94] and the behavioral and autonomic signs observed during spontaneous morphine abstinence.[80,95] These authors suggested, in agreement with the previous clinical results, that the use of clonidine in the detoxification of opiate addicts is based on the suppression of the sympathetic hyperactivity rather than on symptoms with a more behavioral character. In agreement with the non-involvement of central[17] mediated behavioral mechanisms, clonidine was reported to be most effective in reducing withdrawal after peripheral administration than after local central injection.[75] Furthermore, α_2 agonists that do not readily penetrate the blood-brain barrier were able to reduce some symptoms of opiate withdrawal, supporting a peripheral site of action.[75]

The participation of the noradrenergic system in the anti-withdrawal response of clonidine has also been questioned. Thus, some authors have investigated the effects induced by the micro-injection of clonidine into the locus coeruleus in order to investigate this participation.[75,96] The acute administration of clonidine into the locus coeruleus attenuates several somatic symptoms of morphine withdrawal. However, the results concerning the biochemical changes associated with withdrawal-induced noradrenergic hyperactivity are contradictory. The increase in the levels of MHPG induced during opiate abstinence was not modified in the cortex[96] and was prevented in the hippocampus[75] by the infusion of clonidine into the locus coeruleus. Thus, while the locus coeruleus plays a role in the antiwithdrawal effects of clonidine, the lack of correlation between some biochemical and behavioral responses and the previously reported restricted effects of clonidine to only a subset of withdrawal symptoms in animals and humans suggests that other mechanisms different from α_2-adrenoceptors, and probably different from the noradrenergic system, could also be involved in its effects on the morphine withdrawal syndrome.

Another finding supporting the involvement of α_2-adrenoceptors in opiate dependence was the inhibition of the development of dependence by the co-treatment with the α_2-antagonist yohimbine during chronic morphine administration.[97] The blockade of α_2-adrenoceptors by the repeated administration of yohimbine would increase central NA activity, whereas the activation of opioid receptors by morphine should result in antagonistic effects, i.e., a decrease in NA activity. Such opposing actions could block the development of the adaptive changes responsible for the NA hyperactivity that accompanies the withdrawal syndrome.[97] In agreement with this observation, acute injection of yohimbine before morphine withdrawal induced the opposite effect to the repeated administration, i.e., an increase in the behavioral expression of abstinence.[82] Interestingly, the incidence of jumping, the withdrawal sign not suppressed by acute injection of clonidine, was not modified after repeated treatment with yohimbine.[97]

Various studies have reported adaptive changes on α_2-adrenoceptors after chronic administration of opiates, in agreement with the involvement of these receptors in opiate dependence, but the results obtained are controversial. Thus, a reduction in the number[98,99] and sensitivity[13,98] of rat brain α_2-adrenoceptors has been reported after chronic morphine administration, whereas other authors found no changes[100] or an increase[101] in α_2-adrenoceptor density without changes in sensitivity.[100,101] Factors which might underlie these differences include the dose, dosage form, frequency and duration of morphine administration and the brain structure investigated. Accordingly,[102] in the same study, increases, decreases or no changes in α_2-adrenoceptor binding properties were found in different rat brain areas, depending on the duration of opioid treatment. This suggests that α_2-adrenoceptors are unevenly modulated during morphine treatment but ultimately reach baseline values in almost all the brain regions when morphine dependence has clearly developed.[102] Recently, a decrease in the density of α_2-adrenoceptors was found in the postmortem brain of opiate addicts.[103] This adaptive downregulation of α_2-adrenoceptors, whose activation inhibits NA release, like that of μ-opioid receptors, could represent a heterologous desensitization that would tend to overcome the decreased release of NA associated with chronic administration of opiates.[28] During spontaneous morphine abstinence,[102,104] but not after naloxone-precipitated withdrawal,[102] a marked increase in the number of α_2-adrenoceptors was reported. However, the subsensitivity of presynaptic α_2-adrenoceptors persists, indicating that the changes in the size of the total population of α_2-adrenoceptors is not necessarily correlated with changes in the function of presynaptic α_2-adrenoceptors. Since a large proportion of α_2-adrenoceptor binding sites in the rat brain are postsynaptic rather than presynaptic,[105] it is possible that the increase seen during spontaneous abstinence represents an enhancement in postjunctional α_2-adrenoceptors.[104]

Compounds able to act on the postsynaptic α_1-adrenoceptors have also been reported to modify the behavioral manifestations of the morphine withdrawal syndrome, suggesting that the activation of these receptors by NA could participate in the expression of some components of withdrawal. Thus, the administration of the α_1-antagonists phentolamine and phenoxybenzamine decreased the incidence of some somatic signs of opiate withdrawal,[106] whereas the selective α_1-agonist ST 587 increased the expression of body weight loss during morphine withdrawal.[79] The administration of dapiprazole, another α_1-antagonist, prior to morphine has been reported to block the development of acute opiate dependence.[107]

COMPOUNDS ACTING ON β-ADRENOCEPTORS

The effects of β-adrenoceptor antagonists on opiate withdrawal have been evaluated in both animal and human models. Clinical studies report conflicting results on the effectiveness of propranolol in treating heroin addicts. Early studies showed that propranolol prevented the euphoric effects of heroin and reduced the distressing and enduring craving for narcotics in the postwithdrawal abstinence state[108,109] but did not help in the management of the acute physical withdrawal syndrome. In fact, propranolol, in a series of case histories, curiously precipitated delayed opiate withdrawal-like symptoms in heroin addicts when they subsequently, postpropranolol, used heroin.[108-110] However, later studies showed that propranolol actually slightly attenuated the opiate withdrawal syndrome and could be useful in reducing the methadone dose[111] or as an adjunct to clonidine[112] for opiate detoxification. Other studies found that propranolol had no effect on heroin-induced euphoria or craving for narcotics and neither relieved nor precipitated opiate withdrawal in heroin addicts.[113]

Experimental studies in rodents may have clarified the conflicting clinical data, even if they have produced some contradictory results. Early studies showed that propranolol had no effect on the somatic signs of withdrawal precipitated by opiate antagonists in dependent rats.[106,114,115] However, propranolol and atenolol have been recently reported to reduce all of the somatic signs of both naloxone-precipitated and spontaneous abstinence-induced opiate withdrawal.[116,117] This attenuating effect could be due to the blockade of the noradrenergic hyperactivity caused by the supersensitivity of β-adrenoceptors induced by chronic exposure to the opiate agonists. The discrepancy with earlier studies could be due to the higher effectiveness of β-antagonists in reducing the withdrawal syndrome produced by a moderate degree of opiate dependence. Indeed, the doses of morphine and the severity of the withdrawal syndrome were much higher in the earlier studies. This hypothesis may explain the discrepancies reported in earlier clinical studies where propranolol was unable to reduce the acute phase of physical withdrawal but was useful in reducing a less severe state of postwithdrawal abstinence.[108-110,113] Negative motivational aspects of opiate withdrawal were also attenuated by β-adrenoceptor antagonists. Thus, propranolol and atenolol reduced withdrawal-induced anxiety, as assessed by the conditioned defensive burying paradigm[118] and the conditioned place aversion associated with abstinence.[116]

The effects induced by the antagonists of the different subtypes of β-receptors were distinct. Thus, $β_1$-antagonists blocked both jumping and wet dog shakes, whereas $β_2$-antagonists only suppressed the incidence of wet dog shakes.[117] The effects induced by atenolol, which acts preferentially on peripheral $β_1$-adrenoceptors, suggest that peripheral $β_1$-receptors play an important role in the expression of somatic withdrawal symptoms. In addition, propranolol was much more effective in reducing place aversion than atenolol, indicating the potential participation of central β-adrenoceptors.[116,118] However, atenolol shows a high effectiveness in blocking withdrawal-induced anxiety, suggesting that peripheral sympathetic activation may play a major initiating role in this case, possibly providing the necessary input for the activation of the central nervous system.[118]

Biochemical studies investigating β-adrenoceptor binding properties during opiate dependence have revealed adaptive changes, possibly due to the functional interactions between these adrenoceptors and the μ-opioid receptors,[119] that could explain the effects of β-adrenoceptor antagonists on opiate withdrawal. Thus, chronic morphine treatment has been shown to increase the number and sensitivity of β-adrenoceptors, probably in response to decreased presynaptic noradrenergic activity.[120,121] This adaptive change mainly affects $β_1$-adrenoceptors[121] and is particularly intense in the cerebral cortex.[122] However, this supersensitivity was not correlated with the severity of withdrawal behavior during the acute phase of opiate abstinence.[11] After this acute phase, a desensitization of β-adrenoceptors was observed, which was related to the expression of some late symptoms of abstinence, manifesting a noradrenergic hypoactivity.[122]

INDIRECT ADRENERGIC COMPOUNDS

Several indirect adrenergic agonists and antagonists have been evaluated in the morphine withdrawal syndrome. Indirect adrenergic antagonists have been reported to decrease the expression of morphine withdrawal, in agreement with the hypothesis of the important role played in withdrawal expression by the noradrenergic hyperactivity. Indeed, acute administration of a high dose of debrisoquine, which induces an indirect reduction in noradrenergic activity without itself binding to noradrenergic receptors, decreased both the behavioral manifestation of morphine withdrawal and the changes induced in cortical MHPG levels.[11] However, the results obtained by the administration of indirect adrenergic agonists are complicated and sometimes are in contradiction to those obtained by the use of direct agonists. The injection of the adrenergic agonists ephedrine and phenylpropanolamine, which have indirect as well as direct effects on adrenoceptors, decreased the severity of opiate withdrawal.[123] Results obtained with monoamine oxidase inhibitors are not clear. The inhibition by clorgyline administration of central monoamine oxidase A activity, which preferentially acts on NA, has been reported to decrease morphine withdrawal,[124] whereas the blockade by pargyline of central monoamino oxidase B, which acts preferentially on other monoamines but also on NA, was reported to increase[125,126] or not modify[124] the withdrawal syndrome.

DOPAMINERGIC COMPOUNDS

The effects by the dopaminergic compounds on the expression of physical opiate withdrawal are contradictory and depend on the administration route, the compound and the animal species. When dopaminergic agents were given systemically, most of the studies found an increase in the expression of opiate withdrawal after the activation of DA receptors and a decrease by the blockade of these receptors. Acute administration of several DA agonists such as *d*-amphetamine, apomorphine, cocaine, methylphenidate, and L-dopa enhanced wet-dog shakes and aggressive behavior induced during naloxone-precipitated morphine withdrawal syndrome in rats.[127-129] Withdrawal-induced defensive aggression was also facilitated by DA agonists in mice.[130] However, the administration of the D-1 agonist SKF 38393 has been reported to decrease the display of aggressive behavior in mice during morphine withdrawal. The D-2 agonist quinpirole also inhibited withdrawal-induced aggression, but this effect was not specific since a similar decrease in locomotion was observed.[131] Dopaminergic compounds are also able to modify the development of dependence. Indeed, the repeated administration of the specific D-2 agonist bromocriptine during the chronic exposure to morphine results in an inhibition of the development of opiate dependence.[132]

The systemic acute administration of DA antagonists such as haloperidol and butaclamol has been reported to produce opposite effects to DA agonists, i.e., a decrease in the severity of somatic symptoms and aggressive behavior during morphine withdrawal.[127] Haloperidol has also been reported to decrease the severity of withdrawal syndrome in human heroin addicts.[133] In contrast to these results, haloperidol[134] and the selective D-2 antagonist raclopride[135] have been reported to exacerbate the morphine withdrawal response in guinea pigs. However, other neuroleptics with affinity for D-2 receptors such as remoxipride did not modify the manifestation of opiate withdrawal in this model, suggesting that other mechanisms different from the dopaminergic system could be involved in the effects induced by neuroleptics in guinea pigs.[135]

In contrast to most of the results previously obtained after peripheral administration of dopaminergic agents, recent data showed that activation of D-2 receptors within the nucleus accumbens reduced the severity of naloxone-precipitated morphine withdrawal syndrome, whereas the blockade of accumbal D-2 receptors in morphine-dependent animals precipitated somatic withdrawal symptoms. The activation of accumbal D-1 receptors failed to modify the severity of opiate withdrawal. The results indicate that the dopaminergic system in the nucleus accumbens plays an important role in the expression of the somatic symptoms of opiate withdrawal.[136] However, the administration of opiate antagonists into the nucleus accumbens failed to precipitate the withdrawal syndrome in morphine-dependent rats.[137] Consequently, although the nucleus accumbens probably is not a major site for the initiation of physical opiate withdrawal, it seems to play an important role in regulating circuits that drive somatic and aversive responses of opiate withdrawal.

Studies about the involvement of the dopaminergic system in the rewarding properties of opiates also reported some controversial results.[138] Opiates have been shown to be self-administered directly into the region containing the cell bodies of origin of the mesolimbic dopaminergic system, the ventral tegmental area,[139] as well as in the dopaminergic terminal areas such as the nucleus accumbens.[140] However, the reinforcing effects of opiates in the nucleus accumbens seem to be independent of the dopaminergic system since the 6-hydroxydopamine lesion of the nucleus accumbens did not significantly modify heroin self-administration.[141] A similar negative result was obtained in heroin self-administration and heroin-induced place preference after the blockade of the dopaminergic receptors by the administration of the DA antagonist flupentixol.[142,143] In addition, the administration of haloperidol was unable to modify voluntary oral morphine self-administration in high morphine-preferring rats.[144] However, other authors reported that the dopaminergic system could be important in the place preference produced by opiates since it was successfully reversed by the administration of some DA antagonists such as pimozide, haloperidol and SCH23390[145,146] or by specific lesions of the mesolimbic dopamine system.[147,148] Consequently, two different mechanisms seem to be involved in the reinforcing effects of opiates: a dopamine-dependent mechanism probably located in the ventral tegmental area and a dopamine-independent mechanism that may be localized in the nucleus accumbens.[138]

The binding properties of the DA receptors, as well as the intracellular transduction systems coupled to these receptors, have been shown to be modified by acute and chronic morphine exposure. Acute morphine produces an inhibition that affects predominantly postsynaptic dopamine D-1 receptor efficacy by acting on dopamine-sensitive adenylate cyclase.[149] This effect seems to be mainly mediated by an indirect mechanism through inhibition of GABA release at the level of dopamine cell bodies.[58] At the behavioral level, a supersensitivity to the behavioral responses of the dopaminergic agonist apomorphine has been reported after acute morphine administration.[150] During the chronic administration of opiates, most of the studies found that the binding properties (B_{max} and K_d) of D-1 and D-2 receptors remain unaltered.[151,152] Nevertheless, using the dopaminergic agonist apomorphine, it has been reported that chronic morphine treatment is associated with the development of DA receptor supersensitivity.[153] This increased behavioral response could be due to the supersensitivity of DA-sensitive adenylate cyclase in the nucleus accumbens and striatum of rats that was induced in morphine-dependent rats.[154,155] Some authors also found changes in DA receptor binding properties after chronic morphine administration. Thus, the repeated morphine administration in mice produced a decrease in the number of striatal D-2 receptors with no modification in their affinity, whereas the number and affinity of D-1 receptors remained unchanged. This hyposensitivity of D-2 sites was paralleled by an increase in the amount of their coupled second messenger, cAMP.[156]

During morphine withdrawal, the number of D-1 sites, but not of D-2, was increased in several brain structures including hypothalamus, striatum and spinal cord and decreased in amygdala.[151,152] An increase in the K_d value for D-2 receptors, revealing a decreased affinity, was also found by other authors in some brain structures after withdrawal.[157] However, the behavioral responses to both D-1 and D-2 agonists were enhanced in morphine-abstinent rats.[151,152] Changes reported after morphine withdrawal in intracellular messengers coupled to DA receptors in the striatum were dependent on the temporal patterns of morphine treatment as in the case of DA release. Thus, postsynaptic DA D-1 receptor-stimulated adenylate cyclase appeared to be increased within 1-3 days but was unchanged 3 weeks after chronic morphine administration. In contrast, such an enhanced postsynaptic D-1 receptor efficacy did not occur within 1-3 days following repeated morphine treatment but appeared, in this case, 3 weeks after the last injection.[54] Changes induced 1-3 days after withdrawal are probably due to an increase in the number of stimulatory guanine-nucleotide-binding proteins and a decrease in inhibitory guanine-nucleotide-binding proteins without changes in DA D-1 receptor number or intrinsic adenylate cyclase activity[158] (see chapter 3).

REFERENCES

1. Koob GF, Bloom FE. Cellular and molecular mechanisms of drug dependence. Science 1988; 242:715-723.
2. Vogt M. The concentrations of sympathin in different parts of the central nervous system under normal conditions and after the ad-

ministration of drugs. J Physiol (London) 1954; 123:451-481.

3. Gunne LM. Noradrenaline and adrenaline in the rat brain during acute and chronic morphine administration and during withdrawal. Nature 1959; 184:1950-1951.

4. Gunne LM. Catecholamines and 5-hydroxytryptamine in morphine tolerance and withdrawal. Acta Physiol Scand 1963; 58(Suppl):1-91.

5. Maynert EW, Klingman GI. Tolerance to morphine. I. Effects on catecholamines in the brain and adrenal glands. J Pharmacol Exp Ther 1962; 135:285-295.

6. Sloan JW, Eisenman AJ. Long-persisting changes in catecholamine metabolism following addiction to and withdrawal from morphine. In: Wikler A, ed. The Addictive States. Baltimore: Williams & Wilkins, 1968:96-105.

7. Akera T, Brody TM. The addiction cycle to narcotics in the rat and its relation to catecholamines. Biochem Pharmacol 1968; 17:675-688.

8. Segal M, Deneau GA, Seevers MH. Levels and distribution of central nervous system amines in normal and morphine-dependent monkeys. Neuropharmacology 1972; 11:211-222.

9. Kovacs GL, Acsal L, Tihanyi A et al. Catecholamine utilization in distinct mouse brain nuclei during acute morphine treatment, morphine tolerance and withdrawal syndrome. Eur J Pharmacol 1983; 93:149-158.

10. Crawley JN, Laverty R, Roth RH. Clonidine reversal of increased norepinephrine metabolite levels during morphine withdrawal. Eur J Pharmacol 1979; 57:247-250.

11. Swann A, Elsworth JD, Charney DS et al. Brain catecholamine metabolites and behavior in morphine withdrawal. Eur J Pharmacol 1983; 86:167-175.

12. Laverty R, Roth RH. Clonidine reverses the increased norepinephrine turnover during morphine withdrawal in rats. Brain Res 1980; 182:482-485.

13. Roth RH, Redmond DE Jr. Clonidine suppression of noradrenergic hyperactivity during morphine withdrawal: Biochemical studies in rodents and primates. J Clin Psychiatry 1982; 43:42-46.

14. Funada M, Narita M, Suzuki T et al. Effects of pretreatment with pertussis toxin on the development of physical dependence on morphine. Naunyn Schmiedebergs Arch Pharmacol 1993; 348: 88-95.

15. Charney SD, Redmond E Jr, Galloway MP et al. Naltrexone-precipitated opiate withdrawal in methadone-addicted human subjects: Evidence for noradrenergic hyperactivity. Life Sci 1984; 35: 1263-1272.

16. Montel J, Starke K, Taube HD. Morphine tolerance and depen-

dence in noradrenaline neurons of the rat cerebral cortex. Naunyn Schmiedebergs Arch Pharmacol 1975; 288:415-426.

17. Werling LL, Brown SR, Cox BM. Opioid receptor regulation of the release of norepinephrine in brain. Neuropharmacology 1987; 26:987-996.

18. Brodie ME, Laverty R, McQueen EG. Noradrenaline release from slices of the thalamus of normal and morphine-dependent rats. Naunyn Schmiedebergs Arch Pharmacol 1980; 313:135-138.

19. Bianchi C, Siniscalchi A, Veratti E et al. The effects of morphine on monoamine release and content in guinea pig brain slices. Pharmacol Res Commun 1985; 17:377-384.

20. Frankhuyzen AL, Jansen FP, Schoffelmeer ANM et al. Mu-opioid receptor-mediated inhibition of the release of radiolabelled noradrenaline and acetylcholine from rat amygdala slices. Neurochem Int 1991; 19:543-548.

21. Schoffelmeer ANM, Rice KC, Jacobsen JG et al. Mu-, delta- and kappa-opioid receptor-mediated inhibition of neurotransmitter release and adenylate cyclase activity in rat brain slices: Studies with fentanyl isothiocyanate. Eur J Pharmacol 1988; 154:169-176.

22. Mulder AH, Wardeh G, Hogenboom F et al. Selectivity of various opioid peptides towards delta-, kappa- and mu-opioid receptors mediating presynaptic inhibition of neurotransmitter release in the brain. Neuropeptides 1989; 14:99-104.

23. Werling LL, McMahon SR, Cox BM. Selective tolerance at mu and kappa opioid receptors modulating norepinephrine release in guinea pig cortex. J Pharmacol Exp Ther 1988; 247:1103-1106.

24. Pellegrini-Giampietro DE, Bacciottini L, Carlá V et al. Morphine withdrawal in cortical slices: Suppression by Ca^{2+}-channel inhibitors of abstinence-induced [^{3}H]-noradrenaline release. Br J Pharmacol 1988; 93:535-540.

25. De Vries TJ, Ril GTT, Van der Laan JW et al. Chronic exposure to morphine and naltrexone induces changes in catecholaminergic neurotransmission in rat brain without altering mu-opioid receptor sensitivity. Life Sci 1993; 52:1685-1693.

26. Rossetti ZL, Longu G, Mercuro G et al. Extraneuronal noradrenaline in the prefrontal cortex of morphine-dependent rats: Tolerance and withdrawal mechanisms. Brain Res 1993; 609:316-320.

27. Redmond DE Jr. Studies of the locus coeruleus in monkeys and hypotheses for neuropsychopharmacology. In: Meltzer HY, ed. Psychopharmacology: The Third Generation of Progress. New York: Raven Press, 1987:967-975.

28. Done C, Silverstone P, Sharp T. Effect of naloxone-precipitated morphine withdrawal on noradrenaline release in rat hippocampus in vivo. Eur J Pharmacol 1992; 215:333-336.

29. Silverstone PH, Done C, Sharp T. In vivo monoamine release dur-

ing naloxone-precipitated morphine withdrawal. NeuroReport 1993; 4:1043-1045.

30. Laverty R, Sharman DF. Modification by drugs of the metabolism of 3,4-dihydroxyphenylethylamine, noradrenaline and 5-hydroxytryptamine in the brain. Br J Pharmacol 1965; 24:759-772.

31. Sugrue MF. The effects of acutely administered analgesics on the turnover of noradrenaline and dopamine in various regions of the rat brain. Br J Pharmacol 1974; 52:159-165.

32. Moore KE, McCarthy LE, Borison HL. Blood glucose and brain catecholamine levels in the cat following the injection of morphine into the cerebrospinal fluid. J Pharmacol Exp Ther 1965; 148:169-175.

33. Fennessy MR, Lee JR. Comparison of the dose-response effects of morphine on brain amines, analgesia and activity in mice. Br J Pharmacol 1972; 45:240-248.

34. Segal M, Deneau GA. Brain levels of epinephrine, norepinephrine, dopamine and 5-HT during administration and withdrawal of morphine in monkeys. Fed Proc 1962; 21:327.

35. Puri SK, Lal H. Tolerance to the behavioral and neurochemical effects of haloperidol and morphine in rats chronically treated with morphine or haloperidol. Naunyn Schmiedebergs Arch Pharmacol 1974; 282:155-170.

36. Nakamura K, Kuntzman R, Maggio A et al. Effect of 6-hydroxydopamine on catecholamine concentrations and behavior in the morphine-tolerant rat. J Pharm Pharmacol 1972; 24:484-487.

37. Iwamoto ET, Ho IK, Way EL. Elevation of brain dopamine during naloxone-precipitated withdrawal in morphine-dependent mice and rats. J Pharmacol Exp Ther 1973; 187:558-567.

38. Fukui K, Takagi H. Effect of morphine on the cerebral contents of metabolites of dopamine in normal and tolerant mice: Its possible relation to analgesic action. Br J Pharmacol 1972; 44:45-51.

39. Sharman DF. Changes in the metabolism of 3,4-dihydroxyphenylethylamine (dopamine) in the striatum of the mouse induced by drugs. Br J Pharmacol 1966; 28:153-163.

40. Heinrich U, Lichtensteiger W, Langemann H. Effect of morphine on the catecholamine content of midbrain nerve cell groups in rat and mouse. J Pharmacol Exp Ther 1971; 179:259-267.

41. Tseng LF, Loh HH, Ho IK et al. The role of brain catecholamines in naloxone-induced withdrawal in morphine-dependent rats. Proc West Pharmacol Soc 1974; 17:178-183.

42. Gianutsos G, Hynes MD, Puri SK et al. Effect of apomorphine and nigrostriatal lesions on aggression and striatal dopamine turnover during morphine withdrawal: Evidence for dopaminergic supersensitivity in protracted abstinence. Psychopharmacologia 1974;

34:37-44.

43. Lal H. Narcotic dependence, narcotic action and dopamine receptors. Life Sci 1975; 17:483-495.

44. Nowycky MC, Walters JR, Roth RH. Dopaminergic neurons: Effect of acute and chronic morphine administration on single-cell activity and transmitter metabolism. J Neurol Trans 1978; 42:99-116.

45. Mulder AH, Wardeh G, Hogenboom F et al. Kappa- and delta-opioid receptors differentially inhibit striatal dopamine and acetylcholine release. Nature 1984; 308:278-280.

46. Werling LL, Jacoks HM III, McMahon PN. Regulation of [³H]dopamine release from guinea pig striatum by NMDA receptor/channel activators and inhibitors. J Pharmacol Exp Ther 1990; 255:40-45.

47. Heijna MH, Padt M, Hogenboom F et al. Opioid receptor-mediated inhibition of dopamine and acetylcholine release from slices of rat nucleus accumbens, olfactory tubercle and frontal cortex. Eur J Pharmacol 1990; 181:267-278.

48. Heijna MH, Padt M, Hogenboom F et al. Opioid receptor-mediated inhibition of [³H]dopamine but not of [³H]noradrenaline release from rat mediobasal hypothalmus slices. Neuroendocrinology 1991; 54:118-126.

49. Lubetzki C, Chesselet MF, Glowinski J. Modulation of dopamine release in rat striatal slices by delta opioid agonists. J Pharmacol Exp Ther 1982; 222:435-440.

50. Petit F, Hamon M, Fournié-Zaluski MC et al. Further evidence for a role of delta-opioid receptors in the presynaptic regulation of newly synthesized dopamine release. Eur J Pharmacol 1986; 126:1-9.

51. Ronken E, Van Muiswinkel FL, Mulder AH et al. Opioid receptor-mediated inhibition of evoked catecholamine release from culture of rat ventral mesencephalon and locus coeruleus. Eur J Pharmacol 1993; 230:349-355.

52. Ronken E, Mulder AH, Schoffelmeer ANM. Chronic activation of mu- and kappa-opioid receptors in cultured catecholaminergic neurons from rat brain causes neuronal supersentivity without receptor densensitization. J Pharmacol Exp Ther 1994; 268:595-599.

53. Tjon GHK, De Vries TJ, Wardeh G et al. Long-lasting reciprocal changes in striatal dopamine and acetylcholine release upon morphine withdrawal. Eur J Pharmacol 1993; 235:321-322.

54. Tjon GHK, De Vries TJ, Ronken E et al. Repeated and chronic morphine administration causes differential long-lasting changes in dopaminergic neurotransmission in rat striatum without changing its delta- and kappa-opioid receptor regulation. Eur J Pharmacol 1994; 252:205-212.

55. Di Chiara G, Imperato A. Drugs abused by humans preferentially

increase synaptic dopamine concentrations in the mesolimbic system of freely moving rats. Proc Natl Acad Sci USA 1988; 85:5274-5278.

56. Di Chiara G, Imperato A. Opposite effects of mu and kappa opiate agonists on dopamine release in the nucleus accumbens and in the dorsal caudate of freely moving rats. J Pharmacol Exp Ther 1988; 244:1067-1080.

57. Chesselet MF, Cheramy A, Reisine TD et al. Morphine and delta-opiate agonists locally stimulate in vivo dopamine release in cat caudate nucleus. Nature 1981; 291:320-322.

58. Di Chiara G, North RA. Neurobiology of opiate abuse. Trends in Pharmaceutical Sciences 1992; 13:185-193.

59. Spanagel R, Herz A, Shippenberg TS. The effects of opioid peptides on dopamine release in the nucleus accumbens: An in vivo microdialysis study. J Neurochem 1990; 55:1734-1740.

60. Acquas E, Carboni E, Di Chiara G. Profound depression of mesolimbic dopamine release after morphine withdrawal in dependent rats. Eur J Pharmacol 1991; 193:133-134.

61. Pothos E, Rada P, Mak GP et al. Dopamine microdialysis in the nucleus accumbens during acute and chronic morphine, naloxone-precipitated withdrawal and clonidine treatment. Brain Res 1991; 566:348-350.

62. Acquas E, Di Chiara G. Depression of mesolimbic dopamine transmission and sensitization to morphine during opiate abstinence. J Neurochem 1992; 58:1620-1625.

63. Rossetti ZL, Hmaidan Y, Gessa GL. Marked inhibition of mesolimbic dopamine release: A common feature of ethanol, morphine, cocaine and amphetamine abstinence in rats. Eur J Pharmacol 1992; 221:227-234.

64. Sesak SR, Deutch AY, Roth RH et al. Topographical organization of efferent projections of the medial prefrontal cortex in the rat: An anterograde tract-tracing study with Phaseolus vulgaris leucoagglutinin. J Comp Neurol 1989; 290:213-232.

65. Bunney BS, Aghajanian GK. Dopamine and norepinephrine innervated cells in the rat prefrontal cortex: Pharmacological differentiation using microiontophoretic techniques. Life Sci 1976; 19:1783-1792.

66. Spanagel R, Almeida OFX, Shippenberg TS. Long-lasting changes in morphine-induced mesolimbic dopamine release after chronic morphine exposure. Synapse 1993; 14:243-245.

67. Babbini M, Gaiardi M, Bartoletti M. Persistence of chronic morphine effects upon activity in rats 8 months after ceasing the treatment. Neuropharmacology 1975; 14:611-614.

68. Strosberg AD. Structure, function, and regulation of adrenergic

receptors. Protein Sci 1993; 2:1198-1209.

69. Aghajanian GG, Wang YY. Common alpha-2 and opiate effector mechanisms in the locus coeruleus intracellular studies in brain slices. Neuropharmacology 1987; 26:793-799.

70. Gold MS, Redmond DE, Kleben HD. Clonidine in opiate withdrawal. Lancet 1978; 11:599-602.

71. Jasinski DR, Johnson RE, Kocher TR. Clonidine in morphine withdrawal: Differential effects of signs and symptoms. Arch Gen Psychiatry 1985; 42:1063-1066.

72. Buccafusco JJ, Marshall DC, Tarner RM. A comparison of the inhibitory effects of clonidine and guanfacine on the behavioral and autonomic components of morphine withdrawal in rats. Life Sci 1984; 35:1401-1408.

73. Tseng TF, Loh HH, Wei ET. Effects of clonidine on morphine withdrawal signs in the rat. Eur J Pharmacol 1975; 30:93-99.

74. Britton KT, Svensson T, Schwartz J et al. Dorsal noradrenergic bundle lesions fail to alter opiate withdrawal or suppression of opiate withdrawal by clonidine. Life Sci 1984; 34:133-139.

75. Taylor JR, Elsworth JD, Garcia EJ et al. Clonidine infusions into the locus coeruleus attenuate behavioral and neurochemical changes associated with naloxone-precipitated withdrawal. Psychopharmacology 1988; 96:121-131.

76. Tierney C, Nadaud D, Koenig-Berard E et al. Effects of two α_2 agonists, rilmenidine and clonidine, on the morphine withdrawal syndrome and their potential addictive properties in rats. Am J Cardiol 1988; 61:35D-38D.

77. Kelsey JE, Aranow JS, Matthews RT. Context-specific morphine withdrawal in rats: Duration and effects of clonidine. Behav Neurosci 1990; 104:704-710.

78. Redmond DE Jr, Huang YH. The primate locus coeruleus and effects of clonidine on opiate withdrawal. J Clin Psychiatry 1982; 46:25-29.

79. Van der Laan JW. Effects of α_2-agonists on morphine withdrawal behavior: Potentiation of jumping mediated by α_2-receptors. Naunyn Schmiedebergs Arch Pharmacol 1985; 329:293-298.

80. Van der Laan JW, Van't Land CJ. Chronic infusion of clonidine does not alleviate spontaneous morphine withdrawal symptoms in rats. Psychopharmacology 1992; 108:283-288.

81. Coupar IM. Effect of α_2-adrenoceptor agonists on the expression of morphine withdrawal in rats. Naunyn Schmiedebergs Arch Pharmacol 1992; 345:553-557.

82. Dwoskin LP, Neal BS, Sparber SB. Yohimbine exacerbates and clonidine attenuates acute morphine withdrawal in rats. Eur J Pharmacol 1983; 90:269-273.

83. Sparber SB, Meyer DR. Clonidine antagonizes naloxone-induced

suppression of conditioned behavior and body weight loss in morphine-dependent rats. Pharmacol Biochem Behav 1978; 9:319-325.

84. Kosten TA. Clonidine attenuates conditioned aversion produced by naloxone-precipitated opiate withdrawal. Eur J Pharmacol 1994; 254:59-63.

85. Zigun JR, Bannon MJ, Roth RH. Comparison of two α-noradrenergic agonists (clonidine and guanfacine) on norepinephrine turnover in the cortex of rats during morphine abstinence. Eur J Pharmacol 1981; 70:565-570.

86. DiStefano PS, Brown OM. Biochemical correlates of morphine withdrawal. 2. Effects of clonidine. J Pharmacol Exp Ther 1985; 233:339-344.

87. Freedman JE, Aghajanian GK. Opiate and α_2-adrenoceptor responses of rat amygdaloid neurons: Co-localization and interactions during withdrawal. J Neurosci 1985; 5:3016-3024.

88. Aghajanian GK. Tolerance of locus coeruleus neurons to morphine and suppression of withdrawal response by clonidine. Nature 1978; 276:186-188.

89. Rada P, Pothos E, Mark GP et al. Microdialysis evidence that acetylcholine in the nucleus accumbens is involved in morphine withdrawal and its treatment with clonidine. Brain Res 1991; 561:354-356.

90. Gonzalvez ML, Milanés MV, Martinez-Piñero MG et al. Effects of intracerebroventricular clonidine on the hypothalamic noradrenaline and plasma corticosterone levels of opiate-naive rats and after naloxone-induced withdrawal. Brain Res 1994; 647:199-203.

91. Silverstone PH, Done C, Sharp T. Clonidine but not nifedipine prevents the release of noradrenaline during naloxone-precipitated opiate withdrawal: An in vivo microdialysis study in the rat. Psychopharmacology 1992; 109:235-238.

92. Kamisaki Y, Hamahashi T, Hamada T et al. Presynaptic inhibition by clonidine of neurotransmitter amino acid release in various brain regions. Eur J Pharmacol 1992; 217:57-63.

93. Kimes AS, Bell JA, London ED. Clonidine attenuates increased brain glucose metabolism during naloxone-precipitated morphine withdrawal. Neuroscience 1990; 34:633-644.

94. Ignar RD, Kunhn CM. Effects of specific mu and kappa opiate tolerance and abstinence on hypothalamo-pituitary-adrenal axis secretion in the rat. J Pharmacol Exp Ther 1990; 255:1287-1295.

95. Van der Laan JW, de Groot G. Changes in locomotor activity patterns as a measure of spontaneous morphine withdrawal: No effect of clonidine. Drug Alcohol Depend 1988; 22:133-140.

96. Esposito E, Kruszewska A, Ossowska G et al. Noradrenergic and behavioral effects of naloxone injected into the locus coeruleus of morphine-dependent rats and their control by clonidine. Psychop-

harmacology 1987; 93:393-396.

97. Taylor JR, Lewis VO, Elsworth JD et al. Yohimbine co-treatment during chronic morphine administration attenuates naloxone-precipitated withdrawal without diminishing tail-flick analgesia in rats. Psychopharmacology 1991; 103:407-414.

98. Bartoletti M, Gaiardi M, Gubellini C et al. Cross-tolerance between morphine and clonidine: A study on motility in rats. Neuropharmacology 1989; 28:1159-1162.

99. Smith CB, Hollingsworth PJ, Geer JJ et al. Changes in α_2-adrenoceptor in various areas of the rat brain after long-term administration of "mu" and "kappa" opiate agonists. Life Sci 1983; 33(Suppl. I):369-372.

100. Vicentini LM, Miller RJ, Robertson MJ. Chronic opiate treatment does not modify α_2-adrenergic receptors in rat cerebral cortex, kidney and in the neurotumor cell line NCB20. Eur J Pharmacol 1983; 95:265-270.

101. Hamburg M, Tallman JF. Chronic morphine administration increases the apparent number of α_2-adrenenergic receptors in rat brain. Nature 1981; 291:493-495.

102. Ulibarri I, García-Sevilla JA, Ugedo L. Modulation of brain α_2-adrenoceptor and opioid receptor densities during morphine dependence and spontaneous withdrawal in rats. Naunyn Schmiedebergs Arch Pharmacol 1987; 336:530-537.

103. Gabilondo AM, Meana JJ, Barturen F et al. Mu-opioid receptor and α_2-adrenoceptor agonist binding sites in the postmortem brain of heroin addicts. Psychopharmacology 1994; 115:135-140.

104. Smith CB, Moises HC, Spengler RN et al. Changes in α_2-adrenoceptor number and function in brains of morphine-dependent rats. Eur J Pharmacol 1989; 161:111-119.

105. U'Prichard DC. Biochemical characteristics and regulation of brain α_2-adrenoceptors. Ann N Y Acad Sci 1984; 430:55-59.

106. Cicero TJ, Meyer ER, Bell RD. Effects of phenoxybenzamine on the narcotic withdrawal syndrome in the rat. Neuropharmacology 1974; 13:601-607.

107. Valeri P, Martinelli B, Pimpinella G et al. Effects of dapiprazole, clonidine and yohimbine on the development of dependence and withdrawal behavior in mice. Drug Alcohol Depend 1989; 23:73-77.

108. Grosz HJ. Narcotic withdrawal symptoms in heroin users treated with propranolol. Lancet 1972; 2:564-566.

109. Grosz HJ. Successful treatment of a heroin addict with propranolol: Implications for opiate addiction treatment and research. J Indiana State Med Assoc 1972; 65:505-509.

110. Grosz HJ. Effect of propranolol on active users of heroin. Lancet 1973; 2:612.

111. Hollister LE, Prusmack JJ. Propranolol in withdrawal from opi-

ates. Arch Gen Psychiatry 1974; 31:695-698.

112. Roerich H, Gold MS. Propranolol as adjunct to clonidine in opiate detoxification. Am J Psychiatry 1987; 144:1099-1100.

113. Resnick RB, Kestenbaum RS, Schwartz LK et al. Evaluation of propranolol in opiate dependence. Arch Gen Psychiatry 1976; 33:993-997.

114. Jhamandas K, Sutak M, Bell S. Modification of precipitated morphine withdrawal syndrome by drug affecting cholinergic mechanisms. Eur J Pharmacol 1973; 24:296-305.

115. Chipkin RE, Dewey WL, Harris LS et al. Effect of propranolol on antinociceptive and withdrawal characteristics of morphine. Pharmacol Biochem Behav 1975; 3:843-847.

116. Harris GC, Aston-Jones G. Beta-adrenergic antagonists attenuate somatic and aversive signs of opiate withdrawal. Neuropsychopharmacology 1993; 9:303-311.

117. Funada M, Suzuki T, Sugano Y et al. Role of the β-adrenoceptors in the expression of morphine withdrawal signs. Life Sci 1994; 54:113-118.

118. Harris GC, Aston-Jones G. β-adrenergic antagonists attenuate withdrawal anxiety in cocaine- and morphine-dependent rats. Psychopharmacology 1993; 113:131-136.

119. Van Vliet BJ, Ruuls SR, Drukarch B et al. β-adrenoceptor-sensitive adenylate cyclase is inhibited by activation of opioid receptors in rat striatal neurons. Eur J Pharmacol 1991; 195:295-300.

120. Llorens C, Martres M, Bardry M et al. Hypersensitivity to noradrenaline in cortex after chronic morphine: Relevance to tolerance and dependence. Nature 1978; 274:603-605.

121. Kuriyama K. Central β-adrenergic receptor-adenylate cyclase system and formation of morphine withdrawal syndrome. Trends Pharmacol Sci 1982; 3:473-476.

122. Moises H, Smith C. Changes in cortical β-adrenergic receptor density and neuronal sensitivity to norepinephrine accompany morphine dependence and withdrawal. Brain Res 1987; 400:110-126.

123. Dambisya YM, Wong C-L, Chan K. Effects of sympathomimetic agents on opiate analgesia, tolerance and dependence in mice. Methods Find Exp Clin Pharmacol 1991; 13:239-248.

124. Garzon J, Fuentes JA, Del Rio J. Effect of selective monoamine oxidase inhibitor drugs on morphine tolerance and physical dependence in mice. Neuropharmacology 1979; 18:531-536.

125. Iwamoto ET, Shen F, Loh HH et al. The effects of pargyline on morphine tolerant-dependent rats. Fed Proc 1971; 30:278.

126. Maruyama Y, Hayashi G, Smits SE et al. Studies on the relationship between 5-hydroxytryptamine turnover in brain and tolerance and physical dependence in mice. J Pharmacol Exp Ther 1971;

178:308-316.

127. Puri SK, Lal H. Effect of dopaminergic stimulation or blockade on morphine withdrawal aggression. Psychopharmacology 1973; 32:357-361.

128. Lal H, Numan R. Blockade of morphine withdrawal body shakes by haloperidol. Life Sci 1976; 18:163-168.

129. Hynes MD, McCarten MD, Shearman G et al. Differential reduction of morphine withdrawal body shakes by butaclamol enantiomers. Life Sci 1978; 22:133-136.

130. Kantak K, Miczek K. Social, motor, and autonomic signs of morphine withdrawal: Differential sensitivities to catecholaminergic drugs in mice. Psychopharmacology 1988; 96:468-476.

131. Tidey JW, Miczek KA. Morphine withdrawal aggression: Modification with D_1- and D_2-receptor agonists. Psychopharmacology 1992; 108:177-184.

132. Gomaa AA, Mohamed LH, Ahmed HN. Modification of morphine-induced analgesia, tolerance and dependence by bromocryptine. Eur J Pharmacol 1989; 170:129-135.

133. Karkalas J, Lal H. A comparison of haloperidol with methadone in blocking heroin withdrawal symptoms. Intl J Psychiatry Med 1973; 8:248-251.

134. Chahl LA, Thornton CA, Corliss A. Enhancement by haloperidol of the locomotor response induced by naloxone in morphine-treated guinea pigs. Neurosci Lett 1989; 96:213-217.

135. Brent PJ, Chahl LA. Enhancement of the opiate withdrawal response by antipsychotic drugs in guinea pigs is not mediated by sigma binding sites. Eur J Neuropsychopharmacol 1993; 3:23-32.

136. Harris GC, Aston-Jones G. Involvement of D_2 dopamine receptors in the nucleus accumbens in the opiate withdrawal syndrome. Nature 1994; 371:155-157.

137. Maldonado R, Stinus L, Gold LH et al. Role of different brain structures in the expression of the physical morphine withdrawal syndrome. J Pharmacol Exp Ther 1992; 261:669-677.

138. Koob GF. Drugs of abuse: Anatomy, pharmacology, and function of reward pathways. Trends Pharmacol Sci 1992; 13:177-184.

139. Bozarth MA, Wise RA. Anatomically distinct opiate receptor fields mediate reward and physical dependence. Science 1984; 224:516-517.

140. Goeders NE, Lane JD, Smith JE. Self-administration of methionine enkephalin into the nucleus accumbens. Pharmacol Biochem Behav 1984; 20:451-455.

141. Pettit HO, Ettenberg A, Bloom FE et al. Destruction of dopamine in the nucleus accumbens selectively attenuates cocaine but not heroin self-administration in rats. Psychopharmacology 1984;

84:167-173.

142. Mackey WB, van der Kooy D. Neuroleptics block the positive re-inforcing effects of amphetamine but not of morphine as measured by place conditioning. Pharmacol Biochem Behav 1985; 22: 101-105.

143. Stinus L, Nadaud D, Deminiere JM et al. Chronic flupentixol treat-ment potentiates the reinforcing properties of systemic heroin ad-ministration. Biol Psychiatry 1989; 26:363-371.

144. Borg PJ, Taylor DA. Voluntary oral self-administration in rats: Effect of haloperidol and ondansetron. Pharmacol Biochem Behav 1994; 47:633-646.

145. Bozart MA, Wise RA. Heroin reward is dependent on a dopamin-ergic substrate. Life Sci 1981; 29:1881-1886.

146. Leone P, Di Chiara G. Blockade of D_1 receptors by SCH23390 antagonizes morphine- and amphetamine-induced place preference conditioning. Eur J Pharmacol 1987; 135:251-254.

147. Spyraki C, Fibiger HC, Phillips AG. Attenuation of heroin reward in rats by disruption of the mesolimbic dopamine system. Psychop-harmacology 1983; 79:278-283.

148. Shippenberg TS, Herz A, Spanagel R et al. Conditioning of opioid reinforcement: Neuroanatomical and neurochemical substrates. In: Kalivas PW, Samson HH, eds. The Neurobiology of Drug and Alcohol Addiction. 654th ed. New York: Ann NY Acad Sci 1992:347-356.

149. Heijna MH, Bakker JM, Hogenboom F et al. Opioid receptors and inhibition of dopamine-sensitive adenylate cyclase in slices of rat brain regions receiving a dense dopaminergic input. Eur J Pharmacol 1992; 229:197-202.

150. Martin JR, Takemori AE. Increased sensitivity to dopamine ago-nists following a single dose of morphine or levorphanol in mice. Eur J Pharmacol 1985; 119:75-84.

151. Bhargava HN, Gulati A. Modification of brain and spinal cord dopamine D_1 receptors labeled with [^{3}H]SCH-23390 following morphine withdrawal from tolerant and physically dependent rats. J Pharmacol Exp Ther 1990; 252:901-907.

152. Reddy PL, Veeranna P, Thorat SN et al. Evidence for the super-sensitivity of dopamine D_2 receptors without receptor upregulation in morphine-abstinent rats. Brain Res 1993; 607:293-300.

153. Martin JR, Takemori AE. Chronically administered morphine in-creases dopamine receptor sensitivity in mice. Eur J Pharmacol 1986; 121:221-229.

154. Tirone F, Vigano A, Groppetti A et al. Effects of the desensitiza-tion by morphine of the opiate-dependent adenylate cyclase system in the rat striatum on the activity of the inhibitory regulatory G

protein. Biochem Pharmacol 1988; 37:1039-1045.

155. De Vries TJ, Van Vliet BJ, Hogenboom F et al. Effect of chronic prenatal morphine treatment on mu-opioid receptor-regulated adenylate cyclase activity and neurotransmitter release in rat brain slices. Eur J Pharmacol Mol Pharmacol 1991; 208:97-104.

156. Navarro M, Fernandez-Ruiz JJ, Rodriguez de Fonseca F et al. Modifications of striatal D_2 dopaminergic postsynaptic sensitivity during development of morphine tolerance-dependence in mice. Pharmacol Biochem Behav 1992; 43:603-608.

157. Christie MJ, Overstreet DH. Sensitivity of morphine-tolerant rats to muscarinic and dopaminergic agonists: Relation to tolerance and withdrawal. Psychopharmacology 1979; 65:27-34.

158. Van Vliet BJ, Rijswijk ALCTh, Wardeh G et al. Adaptive changes in the number of Gs and Gi proteins underlie adenylate cyclase sensitization in morphine-treated rat striatal neurons. Eur J Pharmacol Mol Pharmacol 1993; 245:23-30.

CHAPTER 5

NEUROPSYCHOPHARMACOLOGY OF OPIATE DEPENDENCE

INTRODUCTION

Opiate drugs are powerful and widely-used analgesic agents. However, their chronic administration is limited by the development of tolerance, indicated by a lowered responsiveness to the drug, coupled with dependence which is evidenced by a heightened responsiveness to opiate antagonists and disturbances upon withdrawal of drugs. These phenomena result from cellular and molecular mechanisms, considered as adaptive processes that develop in response to repeated administration of the drugs, and persist long after the drug has been cleared from the central nervous system. Two types of mechanisms have been proposed to account for these processes: a within-adaptive system and/or a between-adaptive system.[1-4]

Considering the within-adaptive model for both opioid receptors and endogenous opioid peptides, the first hypothesis was that chronic morphine would downregulate opioid receptors.[5] However, while opioid agonist-induced downregulation of binding sites has been clearly observed in vitro in cell cultures,[6-9] this effect was not always observed in vivo.[10-13] A second hypothesis based on data obtained at the cellular level suggests that there is an involvement of second messenger systems such as a modification of the G-protein subunits G_{ia} and G_{oa} ratio, although this has only been shown in the locus coeruleus and amygdala[14,15] (see chapter 3). A third hypothesis is focused on the effects of chronic morphine treatment on opioid-peptide biosynthesis, mainly characterized by the generation of opioid fragments such as -End 1-27 and -End 1-26 with opiate antagonistic properties.[16-18] However, if such adaptive cellular mechanisms can explain some aspects of tolerance, they fail to account for opiate dependence. Two main considerations support this assumption: first, modest doses of naloxone, an opiate antagonist, do not precipitate a withdrawal syndrome in opiate-naive animals, and second, the dose of naloxone required to trigger a withdrawal syndrome decreases as the degree of opiate dependency increases.[19,20]

Such considerations prompted several groups to consider the "between-adaptive system model" which postulates that the morphine-induced changes in primary drug response neurons are triggered by nonopioid neurotransmitter networks which would produce tolerance and/or dependence.[1-4] This model allows consideration of the role of neuropeptides, generically termed antiopioid substances such as cholecystokinin, FMRFamide, -MSH and MIF-1/Tyr-MIF-1-like peptides.[9,11,21-23] Such a hypothesis implies that: (1) in morphine-treated rats, the central nervous system synthesizes and releases antiopioid neuropeptides acting as part of homeostatic systems to neutralize the effects of the opiate drug, and (2) the cessation of opiate receptor stimulation unmasks the relative excess of antiopioid peptides activity. Thus, endogenous antiopioid neuropeptides may be involved in dependence mechanisms and their hyperactivity responsible, at least in part, for the acute withdrawal syndrome associated with the drug removal.

INVOLVEMENT OF ENDOGENOUS PEPTIDES ACTING AS ANTIOPIATES: ROLE OF THE CHOLECYSTOKININ

Cholecystokinin (CCK), the predominant form in the brain which is the sulfated C-terminal octapeptide (CCK-8),[24] has been one of the neuropeptides proposed to act as an antiopioid. Endogenous CCK plays a role in several physiological functions in the central nervous system by interacting with two different receptors, named CCK-A and CCK-B, which have been characterized by pharmacological[25,26] and biochemical[27-29] techniques and have been recently cloned.[30-32] In rodents, CCK-A receptors are located mainly in peripheral tissues such as the pancreas and in a few regions of the brain, whereas the majority of CCK receptors in brain and spinal cord belong to the B type.[28,33] In accordance with the antiopioid model of tolerance and dependence, endogenous CCK could act as a part of a homeostatic mechanism to attenuate opioid responses during the acute and chronic exposure to opiates.[11] Various studies support this hypothesis, showing that CCK agonists and antagonists are respectively able to antagonize and facilitate several pharmacological and biochemical responses induced by opioids.

The pharmacological interactions between CCK and opioid systems were reported for the first time on antinociceptive studies. Thus, CCK-8 was shown to antagonize the antinociception induced by exogenous[21] and endogenous[34] opioids. Paradoxically, CCK-8 and the related analogue caerulein were also able to produce antinociception when administered at higher doses than those shown to block opioid responses.[35] The administration of CCK antagonists has been widely reported to potentiate opiate antinociception.[36] Studies showing facilitatory effects of CCK antagonists on exogenous[37-40] and endogenous[41-43] opioid-induced antinociception have preferentially employed the tail-flick test, in which the nociceptive response is mainly mediated, but not exclusively, at the spinal level. This positive interaction also occurs in response to mechanical pain produced in the rat by paw pressure,[44,45] but was inconsistently observed in the hot-plate test.[40,42,43,46,47] These results suggest that the spinal cord is a strategic site for endogenous CCK/opioid interactions. Accordingly, electrophysiological studies reported specific CCK-opioid interactions at the level of the dorsal horn,[48,49] and a similar localization of opioid and CCK receptors was revealed in the spinal cord in anatomical studies.[50] CCK-B receptors seem to be predominantly involved in the facilitatory effects produced by CCK antagonists in opioid-induced antinociception[40-43,51] (Fig. 5.1). Nevertheless, some studies have also reported these facilitatory responses after the administration of CCK-A antagonists.[36]

The interactions between CCK and opioids are not limited to nociception, and other opioid-mediated effects like hypothermia,[52] changes in locomotor activity,[41,53-55] excitatory effects in hippocampal neurons[56] and body shaking[57] have been antagonized by CCK-8 or CCK agonists. In addition, CCK-B antagonists were

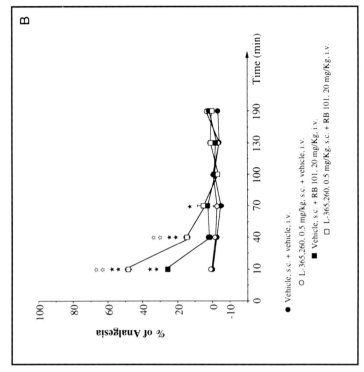

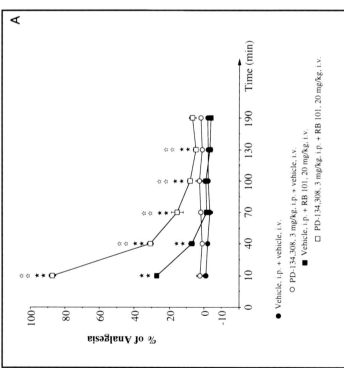

Fig. 5.1. Effects induced by CCK-B antagonists: PD-134,308 (a) and L-365,260 (b) on the antinociceptive responses induced by RB 101, a mixed enkephalin-degrading enzyme inhibitor, in the rat tail-flick. PD-134,308 (3 mg/kg IP) and L-365,260 (0.5 mg/kg SC) were administered 30 minutes before the first tail-flick determination. RB 101 (20 mg/kg IV) was injected 10 minutes before the first tail-flick measurement. Tail-flick latencies were tested at six different times: 10, 40, 70, 100, 130 and 190 minutes after RB 101 injection. The results are expressed as percentages of analgesia ± SEM (n = 8 per group). *p<0.05; **p<0.01 vs vehicle group; white stars vs RB101 group (Schaeffé's F-test). Reproduced with permission from Valverde O et al, Eur J Pharmacol 1995; 286:79-93.

shown to enhance the rewarding properties of morphine in the place-preference test[58,59] and the antidepressant-like effects of endogenous enkephalins in the conditioned suppression of motility paradigm.[60] However, the antagonists of the CCK-A receptors were reported to induce opposite effects, i.e., blockade of the opioid response, in these two behavioral paradigms.[58,60]

The facilitatory effects induced by CCK-B antagonists on endogenous opioid-induced antinociception were blocked by naloxone but were not modified by the δ-opioid antagonist naltrindole, suggesting a selective involvement of μ-opioid receptors.[41,42,61] In contrast, the potentiation observed on endogenous opioid-induced behavioral responses was selectively antagonized by naltrindole, revealing a participation of δ opioid receptors.[60] These results support the existence of a reciprocal modulation between endogenous CCK and opioid pathways, the modification of CCK activity being able to modulate the opioid system but this system, in turn, regulating the release of CCK (Fig. 5.2). Indeed, radioimmunoassay studies have previously reported that morphine administration increases the levels of CCK-8 in the rat.[62]

Biochemical studies also have shown, in vitro and in vivo, differential inhibitory/stimulatory modulation of spinal and supraspinal CCK release by μ- and δ-opioid agonists. Thus, δ opioid activation increases the release of CCK from slices of rat substantia nigra and spinal cord,[63,64] whereas μ opioid agonists suppress CCK release at spinal and supraspinal levels.[63-66] In addition, the in vivo binding of the CCK-B agonist [³H]pBC 264 in rat brain was found to be reduced by administration of RB 101, an inhibitor of the enkephalin catabolism, or of BUBU, a δ-selective agonist, suggesting that endogenous enkephalins increase the extracellular levels of CCK in rodent brains through activation of δ opioid receptors.[67] Consequently, the administration of morphine or the activation of the endogenous opioid system accelerates the release of CCK-8, thereby forming a negative feedback control (Fig. 5.2). Removal of this negative control resulted in an augmentation of the opioid effect. Under physiological conditions, the amount of CCK-8 released seems to be very low,[36] which may explain the fact that CCK receptor blockers do not significantly influence several basal responses, such as nociceptive threshold. The potentiation of opioid-induced pharmacological responses by CCK-B antagonists could be due to modifications in endogenous opioid release, but it could also occur directly by changes in intracellular events. Thus, CCK and opioid receptors, which both belong to the group of G-protein-coupled binding sites,[31] are co-localized on the same neurons in discrete areas of rat brain,[68,69] and an improvement of the intracellular transduction mechanisms associated with opioid receptor stimulation could result from CCK-B receptor blockade.

This hypothetical model of reciprocal interactions between the endogenous CCK and endogenous opioid systems has been postulated from the acute responses obtained in pharmacological and biochemical studies. Nevertheless, it could also explain the interactions occurring between these two systems during the chronic administration of opiates. Thus, the development of tolerance to the antinociceptive effects that appears after chronic morphine administration was prevented by the repeated injection of CCK-A or CCK-B antagonists, which given alone did not modify the nociceptive threshold.[70-75] CCK-B receptors seem to be predominantly involved in this effect.[75] Tolerance to morphine was also reversed by the administration of antiserum against CCK-8, whereas anti-

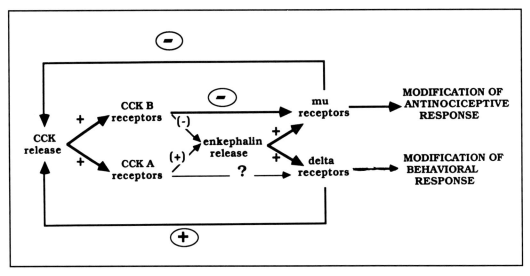

Fig. 5.2. Hypothetical model of the reciprocal interactions between the endogenous CCK system and the endogenous opioid system. Reproduced with permission from Maldonado R et al, Neuro Report 1993; 7:947-950.

serum per se did not produce any effect on antinociception, nor did it affect the acute antinociception induced by morphine.[74] Consequently, tolerance development may result, at least in part, from a progressive compensatory increase in the activity of endogenous CCK systems in response to prolonged opiate administration. This increased activity would be counteracted by the administration of CCK antagonists or CCK antiserum. This hypothesis is supported by recent biochemical findings reporting that the repeated morphine administration produces a compensatory increase in CCK mRNA in several brain structures including hypothalamus, spinal cord, brain stem[76] and amygdala.[77] Furthermore, an upregulation of the mRNA for CCK was observed in sensory neurons of rat lumbar dorsal root ganglia after unilateral sectioning of the sciatic nerve. This increase could be associated with a release of CCK from primary afferent terminals, inducing morphine insensitivity. Morphine antinociceptive response was re-established in this experimental neuropathic model by the administration of a CCK-B antagonist.[51]

In spite of the involvement of CCK in the development of opiate tolerance, the role of endogenous CCK in opiate dependence is not clear. Thus, the repeated injection of nonspecific CCK antagonists, such as proglumide and benzotript, or specific CCK-A (devazepide) and CCK-B (L-365,260) antagonists did not modify the expression of the somatic symptoms of withdrawal precipitated by naloxone in morphine-dependent rats.[37,72,73,75] Furthermore, the acute administration of the CCK-B antagonist PD-134,308 before naloxone did not modify the somatic manifestations of morphine abstinence.[78] PD-134,308, which has no affinity for opioid binding sites,[79] was found to slightly inhibit the in vivo binding of [³H]diprenorphine, suggesting that this CCK-B antagonist facilitates the release of endogenous opioids. However, the increase in endogenous enkephalin levels was probably not strong enough to modify the severity of withdrawal syndrome in accordance with the small magnitude of the biochemical response found in this in vivo binding study.[78] Even if acute or chronic administrations of CCK antagonists were unable to modify the expression of opiate abstinence, PD-134,308 strongly potentiated the antiwithdrawal effects induced by the inhibitor of the enkephalin catabolism

RB101,[78] as discussed in chapter 7. This effect was presumably due to the facilitatory actions of the CCK antagonist on the acute response induced by RB101.

Another approach to investigate the participation of the CCK system in opiate dependence consisted of evaluating the ability of different CCK agonists to induce behavioral signs of withdrawal after acute injection in morphine-dependent animals and comparing this response to that produced by the administration of an opiate antagonist. The peripheral administration of CCK-8 did not precipitate any sign of withdrawal after morphine chronic treatment, but the failure of CCK-8 to precipitate withdrawal could be due to its inability to cross the blood brain barrier.[80] In order to investigate the specific role of the central CCK system on the expression of opiate dependence, the effects produced by the intracerebroventricular injection of different CCK agonists were also evaluated by using this experimental procedure.[81] Central administration of a selective CCK-B agonist, BC264,[82] induced a strong and dose-dependent increase in locomotor activity and rearing behavior in morphine-dependent animals. This response was not due to an intrinsic effect of BC264 since it was observed with doses that did not modify locomotion in saline control animals. CCK-8 produced a slight effect on these behavioral responses, which was only observed after the administration of moderate doses (1 µg), but not when lower or higher doses were injected.[81] The higher effectiveness of BC264 indicates a selective participation of CCK-B receptors. The lack of effect following administration of a high dose of CCK-8 could be due to an opposite effect of CCK-A and CCK-B receptor stimulation, in agreement with the opposite role played by these two CCK receptors on other pharmacological responses.[60,83]

Several hypotheses may explain the behavioral changes induced by CCK agonists, particularly by BC264, after chronic morphine treatment. Indeed, the administration of the CCK-B agonist in morphine-dependent rats only induced nonspecific signs of withdrawal, such as increases in locomotor activity and rearing behavior. The hyperactivity induced by BC264 might be, first, the result of a selective interaction on locomotor activity. However, this hypothesis seems unlikely since BC264 did not increase activity in animals receiving an acute injection of different doses of morphine; on the contrary, it decreased morphine-induced hyperactivity.[81] Both CCK-B receptor activation by BC264 and blockade of opioid receptors by naloxone induced a similar hyperactivity in morphine-dependent rats. Consequently, a second hypothesis is that this hyperactivity may reflect an antiopioid effect induced by the CCK-B agonist, i.e., the expression of a mild morphine withdrawal syndrome. Thus, the activation of CCK receptors could be not enough to induce the presence of major withdrawal signs in morphine-dependent rats, but it could be sufficient enough to induce the presence of some minor signs such as the increase in locomotion and rearing behavior.[81] Whatever the significance of these behavioral changes, the role played by the CCK system on the expression of physical opioid dependence seems to be minor.

However, the interaction between CCK and the expression of the motivational aspects of morphine dependence has not been elucidated. Physical and motivational components of opiate withdrawal involve different neural pathways: locus coeruleus and mesolimbic systems, respectively.[84] Considering the role played by CCK on the control of emotional states[85,86] and the involvement of the mesolimbic system in this effect,[26] it would be possible that the changes observed in locomotion could be associated with the expression of other motivational aspects of morphine dependence. Further studies need to be performed in order to clarify this point.

INVOLVEMENT OF ENDOGENOUS PEPTIDES ACTING AS ANTIOPIATES: ROLE OF NEUROPEPTIDE FF

The neuropeptide Phe-Leu-Phe-Gln-Phe-Gln-Arg-Phe-NH2 (NPFF), previously called F8Fa, was detected in mammalian brain through its cross-reaction with an antibody directed to the molluscan cardioactive tetrapeptide Phe-Met-Arg-Phe-NH2 (FMRF-NH2)[87,88] and was later isolated from bovine brain.[23] Extensive NPFF immunoreactivity has been reported in the CNS of the rat, with the highest concentrations occurring in the spinal cord, hypothalamus, pons-medulla and neural lobe of the pituitary.[89-92] In addition, specific receptors to NPFF have been demonstrated in rat CNS via binding studies, with the highest densities occurring in the spinal cord, periaqueductal gray matter, thalamus, amygdala and lateral septum.[93,94] Although the exact physiological role of NPFF remains to be established, there are several reasons to hypothesize that NPFF is an endogenous peptide with antiopiate activities. Intracerebroventricular (ICV) injection of FMRF-NH2- and NPFF-related peptides attenuate morphine- and stress-induced analgesia[23,70,95-98] and morphine-induced eating.[99] IgG prepared from NPFF antiserum increases both morphine- and stress-induced analgesia[100] and reverses morphine tolerance.[101] An NPFF antagonist has similar effects.[102] Acute administration of morphine releases FMRF-NH2 immunoreactivity from rat spinal cord,[103] chronic ICV infusion of NPFF downregulates μ opioid binding sites in rat brain,[104] and NPFF attenuates the inhibition of spinal cord C-fiber-evoked activity resulting from intrathecal administration of a μ opioid receptor agonist.[105] Interestingly, this study showed also that NPFF does not attenuate the inhibition of spinal cord C-fibers-evoked activity resulting from intrathecal administration of a δ opioid receptor agonist, suggesting that, at least in the spinal cord, NPFF exhibits receptor selectivity (Fig. 5.3).

Several results also postulate the involvement of NPFF-like peptides in opiate dependence. The ICV injection of NPFF induced a morphine-reversible quasi-abstinence syndrome in opiate-naive rats,[106] while either ICV administration of NPFF antiserum[107] or injection of a NPFF antagonist[108] both attenuated a naloxone-precipitated withdrawal syndrome in morphine-dependent rats. The hypothesis of the direct involvement of NPFF hyperactivity has been confirmed by biochemical approaches. Chronic morphine treatment (subcutaneous implantation of slow-release morphine pellets) has recently been shown to induce activation of NPFF neuronal activity which parallels the establishment of tolerance and dependence to opiates[109] (Fig. 5.4). Polyphasic modifications of neuropeptide FF immunoreactivity (NPFF-IR) have been reported in hypothalamus, brain stem, and cervical and thoracolumbar areas, consisting first of a rapid decrease (-52%) of NPFF-IR between 1-2 hours postimplant, followed by a dramatic increase (+127%) that reached a maximum between 3-12 hours postimplant and a return to the control values at the end of the first day. It is likely that a dramatic increase in NPFF release may account for the initial reduction of NPFF-IR levels, not yet compensated by

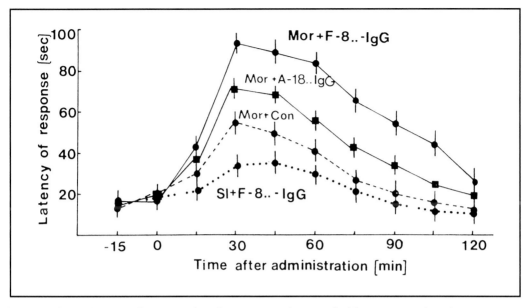

Fig. 5.3. Effects of intracerebroventricular administration of IgG purified from F8F-NH2 (NPFF) or A18F-NH2 antisera on morphine-induced analgesia in single mice (hot plate, morphine, 10 mg/kg). Mor + F8F IgG group; Mor + A18F IgG group; and control groups, respectively, Mor + Con which received morphine and saline ICV, and SI + F8 IgG which received saline and F8F-NH2 antibody ICV. Reproduced with permission from Kavaliers M et al, Peptides 1989; 10:741-745.

peptide or precursor biosynthesis at the level of the cell bodies. Thus, the activity of these NPFF-IR neurons may increase gradually as a consequence of the continuous stimulation of opiate receptors, inducing a compensatory increase in peptide synthesis and transport processes which could transiently exceed NPFF-IR release (Fig. 5.5). The transient increase in NPFF-IR content, observed between 3-12 hours post-pellet implantation, may be an indication of this imbalance state. The return to the basal level of endogenous NPFF-IR could be the result of the match of an increased release compensated by an increased synthesis of NPFF as part of a homeostatic process. Therefore, since the delay to observe the total disappearance of morphine-induced analgesia was 36 hours post-implant, one could postulate that this is the time required for antiopiate systems to achieve a sufficient level of activity to counteract morphine analgesic effects. These results and this hypothesis are in agreement with the 2-fold increase of

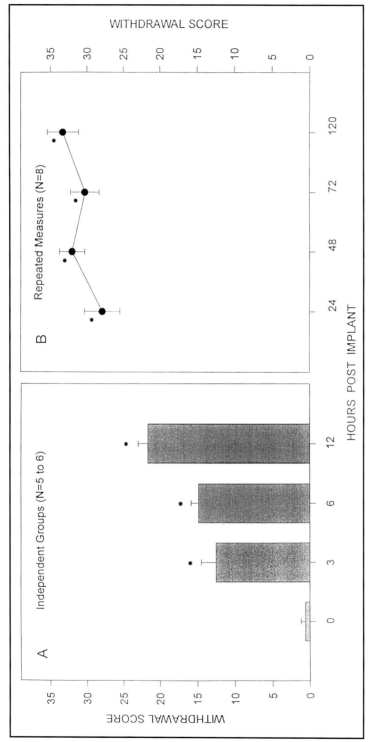

Fig. 5.4. Time course of opiate dependence following morphine pellet implantation. Withdrawal score (SEM) was evaluated using the Gellert-Holtzman scale during 10 minutes following naloxone injection (1 mg/kg SC). The left panel (A) indicates the withdrawal score 3, 6 and 12 hours postimplantation measured in independent groups of rats (n = 6 each). The right panel (B) shows naloxone-induced opiate withdrawal measured 24, 48, 72 and 120 hours postimplantation in a separate group of eight rats with repeated measures. *p<0.01 when compared to placebo implanted rats (n = 5) tested at either 3, 6 or 12 hours postimplantation and which data were plotted and represented by delay 0 hour. Reproduced with permission from Stinus L et al, Peptides 1995; 16:1235-1241.

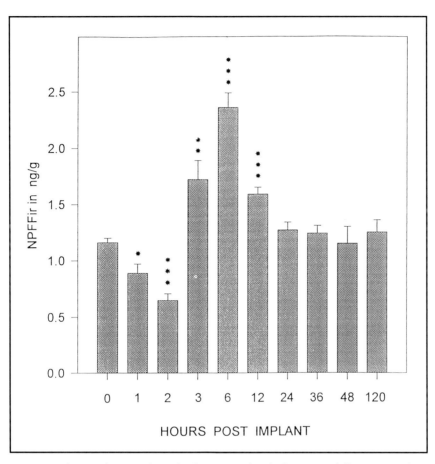

Fig. 5.5. Evolution of NPFF-IR (in ng/g of tissue SEM) in the brain stem following morphine pellet implantation (n = 12 or 24 rats). Control rats were implanted with placebo pellets and sacrificed at the same intervals as morphine-implanted rats. Control rats' data were pooled and plotted as one group (n = 132) designated as 0 hour postimplantation. ***p<0.001, **p<0.01, *p<0.05 when compared with placebo-pelleted rats. Reproduced with permission from Stinus L et al, Peptides 1995; 16:1235-1241.

NPFF-IR previously reported in CSF collected from 7-day morphine-dependent rats[107] (Table 5.1).

The exact cellular mechanisms by which opiate receptor stimulation activates the antiopioid system is still unclear. However, it has been recently proposed that NMDA receptors may be important in the development of opiate tolerance and dependence,[110] and it has been shown that glutamate triggers NPFF-IR release from rat spinal cord slices via NMDA receptors.[111]

Table 5.1. F8F-NH-2 (NPFF) immunoactivity in CFS

n	CSF Source	F8F-NH$_2$ Immunoreactivity (pmol/ml)
Pooled CSF Samples:		
7	Saline-infused rats	0.053 pmol/ml
7	Morphine-infused rats	0.097 pmol/ml

n	CSF Source	F8F-NH$_2$ Immunoreactivity (Mean SEM)
Individual CSF Samples:		
21	Saline-infused rats	0.057 ± 0.014 pmol/ml
21	Morphine-infused rats	$0.104 \pm 0.020^*$ pmol/ml

* p<0.05 vs. saline
Following 7 days of continuous peripheral infusion of morphine with Alzet osmotic minipumps (1.5 mg/kg/hour). Reproduced with permission from Malin DH et al, Peptides 1990; 11:969-972.

Together, these results support the initial hypothesis that the development of tolerance to the analgesic effects of opiates could be parallel and functionally linked to the gradual increase of the activity of antiopiate neuronal networks such as NPFF or CCK. It could explain why administration of IgG from antiserum against NPFF-IR or antagonists of CCK, another putative antiopioid peptide, may prevent or reverse the development of tolerance in morphine-treated rats.[37,71,101,112] It suggests that the clinical use of a putative antagonist of NPFF receptors in association with morphine may not only protect against tolerance but also potentiate morphine-induced pain relief.

INVOLVEMENT OF ENDOGENOUS PEPTIDES ACTING AS ANTIOPIATES: ROLE OF DYNORPHIN

Dynorphin is an opioid peptide which is thought to be the endogenous ligand for the κ-opioid receptor. In addition to producing κ-agonist effects, dynorphin acts as a μ-antagonist.[113] There is compelling evidence that dynorphin functions as part of an antiopioid system. Dynorphin negatively modulates morphine- and β-endorphin-induced antinociception.[114] Intrathecal administration of dynorphin (1-17) attenuates morphine-induced analgesia, while anti-dynorphin (1-17) antibodies potentiate this effect.[115-117] The acute tolerance which develops in response to a single large dose of morphine is mediated in part by spinal dynorphin (1-17) mechanisms.[118] Nor-binaltorphimine (nor-BNI) produces α κ-receptor blockade which persists for at least 1 month in the rat.[119] In morphine-dependent rats, the ICV injection of nor-BNI potentiates naloxone-induced place aversion and behavioral measures of naloxone-precipitated withdrawal and enhances the reduction of basal mesolimbic dopamine release recorded during opiate withdrawal which may contribute to aversive or dysphoric states associated with opiate withdrawal.[120] These findings are in line with those of other studies suggesting that inactivation of endogenous κ-opioid systems may exacerbate the naloxone-precipitated withdrawal signs in morphine-dependent rats and mice.[121,122] Thus, dynorphin may act as a functional antagonist of the mood-enhancing effects of morphine.

PARTICIPATION OF DIFFERENT BRAIN STRUCTURES IN THE EXPRESSION OF OPIATE WITHDRAWAL

Chronic administration of opiates induces physical dependence, which is characterized by a withdrawal syndrome associated with the disruption of the narcotic treatment or with the administration of an opioid antagonist. This withdrawal syndrome is manifested by a variety of specific autonomic, behavioral and motivational symptoms. Several approaches have been followed to evaluate the anatomical brain sites involved in the expression of the different manifestations of opiate abstinence. Each one of these approaches has some precise limitation and weakness, but taken together, all results led to the identification, in most cases, of the specific role played by the different brain structures. One of the methods currently used consists of making animals physically dependent by systemic administration of opiates and precipitating a withdrawal syndrome by local central administration of a narcotic antagonist in a specific brain structure. Opioid antagonists currently used in these studies, such as naloxone or naltrexone, have high lipophilic properties. In order to address the problem of extensive drug spread with the local administration of a lipophilic opioid antagonist, several authors used crystalline naloxone application to reduce the diffusion of the drug from the liquid injection.[123,124]

However, it has been shown that crystalline drug application can also result in a great and rapid diffusion which may be due to the extremely high concentration of drug applied with this method.[125] For instance, in the case of dopamine, less diffusion was seen after liquid[126] than crystalline[125] application. Others have used hydrophilic opiate antagonists, like methylnaloxonium, which have been shown to considerably reduce the diffusion out of the region into which the drug is injected. Thus, labeled methylnaloxonium was found to remain at the site of injection much longer than labeled naloxone (10 minutes versus 60 minutes, respectively).[127] Consequently, the response observed after the local injection of this hydrophilic antagonist in one brain structure may be more selective than that obtained with the application of lipophilic antagonists.

A second approach is to investigate the effects of a chemical or electrolytic lesion of a brain structure on the development of opiate dependence. The results obtained by using this method have been contradictory in many of the reports, and they differ depending on the procedure used and the extent of the lesion. In addition, neuronal adaptive mechanisms can develop after a brain lesion in order to compensate for any deficits in physiological function. These compensatory mechanisms can be very complex and make difficult the interpretation of the results from lesion studies. Another approach involves the direct intracranial application of morphine into specific brain sites. Apart from the problem of drug diffusion, the main limitation of this method is that the level of tissue damage after chronic morphine infusion was higher than that usually seen in studies using a similar infusion volume over a shorter time interval (Bozarth, unpublished observations; cited in Bozarth, 1984[128]).

The results obtained by using these three approaches have generally supported the hypothesis that no single brain structure is responsible for the expression of opiate withdrawal syndrome, suggesting a widespread brain distribution for this neuroanatomical substrate. Intracerebral injections of opiate antagonists identified several brain regions implicated in the expression of the different components of morphine abstinence. The locus coeruleus and, in a second order, the periaqueductal gray matter were the structures most sensitive to opiate antagonist-precipitated morphine physical withdrawal syndrome.[129] Mesolimbic structures, and particularly the nucleus accumbens, were the most sensitive in the precipitation of negative motivational aspects of opiate withdrawal.[130,131] Lesion studies have confirmed the crucial role played by the locus coeruleus in the expression of the somatic symptoms of opiate abstinence.[132] However, when opiate agonists were directly perfused into different brain areas, the most severe degree of opiate dependence was induced within or in the proximity of the periaqueductal gray matter.[128] The relevance of all these results and the role that has been proposed for each different brain structure will be discussed in this section.

LOCUS COERULEUS

The locus coeruleus is the largest cluster of noradrenergic neurons in the brain[133,134] and represents the primary source of noradrenergic innervation of the limbic system, cerebral and cerebellar cortices, and a quantitatively smaller source of innervation of hypothalamic, spinal cord and other brain stem nuclei.[135] Multiple receptors, including opioid and noradrenergic receptors, seem to converge onto single effectors and to exert a synergistic action in this brain structure.[136] One of the first pieces of evidence suggesting the involvement of this brain structure in the expression of the somatic symptoms of opioid withdrawal was the observation that the electrical stimulation of the locus coeruleus produces several behavioral and physiological signs that are similar to the opiate abstinence syndrome in opiate-naive monkeys.[137-140] These signs were blocked by decreasing noradrenergic activity by the administration of the α_2-adrenergic agonist clonidine.[139]

The effects induced by acute and chronic opiate treatment on the spontaneous firing of noradrenergic neurons in the locus coeruleus also support the participation of this structure in the expression of morphine withdrawal. The acute injection of opioid agonists induces an inhibition of noradrenergic neurons firing in the locus coeruleus.[141] A tolerance was observed to this response, shown by a reduction in the sensitivity of locus coeruleus neurons to the inhibitory effect induced by the opioids.[142] The administration of an opioid antagonist in dependent animals induced a withdrawal response in the locus coeruleus revealed by a rebound hyperactivity, i.e., an increase in the noradrenergic neuron firing rate.[143,144] Abstinence to opiates was also demonstrated in this noradrenergic structure by an enhancement in the turnover of noradrenaline,[145] levels of 3-methoxy-4-hydroxy-phenethyleneglycol (MHPG)[146] and tyrosine-hydroxylase activity.[147] Chronic morphine treatment and withdrawal induce large changes in the locus coeruleus in second messenger systems coupled to opioid receptors. Indeed, chronic morphine administration has been reported to upregulate the cAMP pathway in the locus coeruleus, but not in several other brain regions such as neostriatum, frontal cortex and dorsal raphe.[148] This process includes adaptive changes in cAMP-dependent protein kinase, adenylate cyclase, G proteins, cAMP-regulated phosphoproteins and cAMP response element-binding protein phosphorylation.[14] A striking parallel between changes in some of these parameters (increased level of G-proteins and upregulation of the cAMP system), the time course of behavioral abstinence symptoms and the increase in the firing rates of the locus coeruleus noradrenergic neurons was observed during antagonist-precipitated morphine withdrawal.[149] The molecular changes in cAMP cascade and its relevance to the development and expression of opiate dependence are addressed in chapter 3.

The locus coeruleus was the most sensitive site to precipitate withdrawal syndrome in morphine-dependent rats by the local administration of the hydrophilic opiate antagonist methylnaloxonium[129] (Fig. 5.6). Thus, an elevated frequency of the majority of the somatic symptoms of withdrawal was observed, and the expression of the motor component of the abstinence (jumping, rearing and hyperactivity) was particularly intense. Moreover, animals with the final site of injection outside of but in proximity to the locus coeruleus exhibited a lower severity of the abstinence. In agreement with this observation, a morphine behavioral abstinence associated with increased concentrations of MHPG in the cerebral cortex was also observed after local injection of naloxone in the locus coeruleus of dependent rats.[150] Furthermore, the withdrawal syndrome induced by the administration into the lateral ventricle of methylnaloxonium in animals with a partial or a full electrolytic lesion of the locus coeruleus was less severe than that induced in sham-operated animals, providing further evidence that

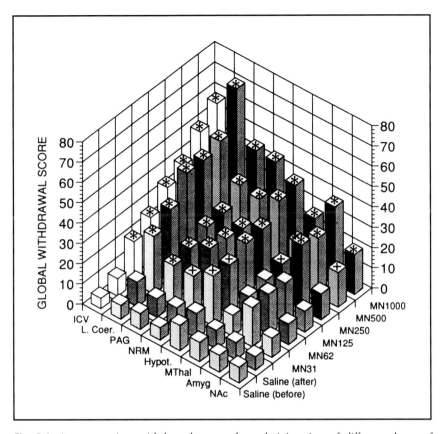

Fig. 5.6. Average opiate withdrawal score after administration of different doses of methylnaloxonium in different brain structures. The z-axis represents the different treatments: saline (before) shows the control performed before methylnaloxonium injections; saline (after) expresses the control performed at the end of the experimental sequence (doses of methylnaloxonium are expressed in nanograms). The x-axis represents the different brain structures where the methylnaloxonium was administered: ICV, lateral ventricle; L.Coer., locus coeruleus; PAG, periaqueductal gray matter; NRM, nucleus raphe magnus; Hypot., anterior hypothalamus; MThal., medial thalamus; Amyg, central amygdala; NA₀, nucleus accumbens. The y-axis expresses the values of the means for each column (n = 6 per group). White columns represent animals injected with methylnaloxonium ICV. Shaded columns express groups of animals treated with methylnaloxonium in other brain structures. $^{+}p<0.05$ and $^{*}p<0.01$ indicate that the group was different from the two saline controls performed in the corresponding brain structure (Newman-Keuls test). Reproduced with permission from Koob GF et al, Trends Neurosci 1992; 15:186-191.

the integrity of the locus coeruleus is important for the development and manifestation of physical opiate dependence in rats.[132] Electrolytic lesion of the medial noradrenergic forebrain bundle also reduced the somatic expression of opiate abstinence. This effect was observed when a severe degree of dependence was induced, but did not appear when morphine was administered for a shorter period of time, inducing only a moderate degree of dependence.[151] However, the results obtained after catecholaminergic depletion induced by the administration of 6-hydroxydopamine (6-OHDA) are controversial. Thus, the 6-OHDA lesion of the dorsal noradrenergic bundle originating into the locus coeruleus failed to alter the severity of morphine withdrawal.[152] These discrepancies could be due to the less widespread depletion obtained after 6-OHDA lesion than with electrolytic lesion (Fig. 5.7).

Indeed, the NA levels in the cerebellum were not modified after 6-OHDA lesions,[152] whereas the electrolytic lesion of the locus coeruleus produced a significant depletion. Consequently, it is possible that some noradrenergic fibers, such as the pontine or descending projections of the locus coeruleus, are critically involved in the expression of the withdrawal syndrome and remained untouched after the 6-OHDA lesion. Consistent with this hypothesis, several reports suggest that the spinal sympathetic preganglionic neurons may contribute to the expression of morphine abstinence.[153-156] When 6-OHDA was administered in order to reach the whole brain, the effects on morphine withdrawal seemed to be due to a denervation supersensitivity induced by the neurotoxin, and they are opposite to those obtained after the electrolytic lesion of the locus coeruleus.

Indeed, both intracerebral injection of 6-OHDA in mice[157] and its intracisternal administration in two-week-old rats[158] exacerbated the behavioral expression of the morphine withdrawal syndrome. These responses were specific for NA depletion since in both cases an approximately 66% depletion of NA was observed, and the effects did not appear when desmethylimipramine was administered prior to 6-OHDA in order to preferentially deplete dopamine.[158] Rats treated with 6-OHDA undergoing withdrawal had higher levels of NA than the corresponding control/depleted animals,[158] which could reflect an increase in NA release in spite of the neurotoxin injection. Consequently, the exacerbation of physical dependence might be due to this increase in NA release, which would induce a strong noradrenergic hyperactivity as a consequence of the postsynaptic supersensitivity induced by 6-OHDA. A recent study reported that the intracerebral administration of the noradrenergic

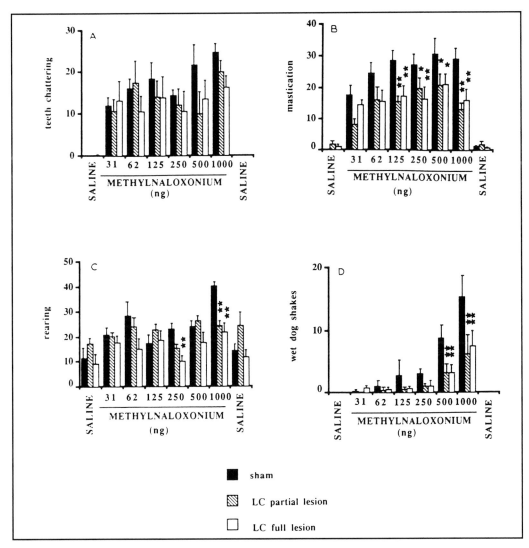

Fig. 5.7. Effects of locus coeruleus electrolytic lesions on the different signs of morphine withdrawal syndrome (a: teeth chattering, b: mastication, c: rearing, d: wet dog shakes) after ICV administration of methylnaloxonium. Abscissa represents the different doses: saline group placed at the left shows the control vehicle injection performed before the injection of methylnaloxonium; saline group placed at the right shows the control vehicle injection performed after methylnaloxonium injection. Numbers on the ordinate express the values of the mean ± SEM for each group (n = 6-8 per group). *p<0.05; **p<0.01 main overall lesion effect ANOVA with significant overall difference between both lesion groups and the sham group (Newman-Keuls test). Reproduced with permission from Maldonado R et al, Brain Res 1993; 605:128-138.

neurotoxin DSP-4, which selectively damages NA-containing nerve endings, strongly decreased the severity of naloxone-precipitated morphine withdrawal.[159] However, in this experiment the denervation supersensitivity was probably not developed since the neurotoxin was injected only 24 hours before withdrawal syndrome, and NA depletion was less than 30%.

In contrast with the results obtained by administering opiate antagonists, the physical dependence produced by morphine infusions into the caudal part of the periaqueductal gray matter, into the vicinity of the locus coeruleus, was less severe than that induced by infusions into the rostral part of the periaqueductal gray matter. An elevated incidence of some signs such as teeth chattering and wet dog shakes was observed, but the level of jumping was less intense.[160] The level of tissue damage after chronic infusion has been reported to be higher than after acute injection of a compound (Bozarth, unpublished observations; cited in Bozarth, 1984[128]). Consequently, taking into account the small size of the locus coeruleus, the discrepancies between these results could be due to the possible damage induced in this structure and/or some of its projections by the chronic opiate administration procedure.

Recent studies using in situ hybridization have also emphasized the role played by the locus coeruleus in opioid dependence. Thus, type VIII adenylate cyclase mRNA was selectively increased after chronic morphine treatment in the locus coeruleus, and the time course of these changes in adenylate cyclase mRNA was related to the incidence of jumping behavior during the withdrawal syndrome.[161] Another argument in favor of the role of this intracellular signal transduction pathway is the strong attenuation in the expression of the somatic symptoms of morphine withdrawal that results from the inhibition of protein kinase activity into the locus coeruleus.[162] Protein kinases belonging to the family of the serine/threonine kinases seem to be selectively implicated since this reduced withdrawal response was induced by the local administration of the serine/threonine kinase inhibitor H7, but not after the microinjection of the tyrosine kinase inhibitor KB23.[162]

The important role of the locus coeruleus in the expression of the somatic symptoms of abstinence suggested by all these studies may explain the mild withdrawal syndrome observed after the chronic administration of inhibitors of enkephalin catabolism[163,164] since no demonstration of synaptic responses to endogenously released opioids has been reported in this region. Indeed, the administration of inhibitors of the enkephalin-degrading enzymes had no effect of their own on the properties of locus coeruleus neurons, suggesting that the tonic and synaptically evoked release of endogenous opioids in the locus coeruleus is weak.[165]

Nucleus Paragigantocellularis

The activation of noradrenergic neuron firing in the locus coeruleus induced by systemically administered opiate antagonists to morphine-dependent animals was not observed in isolated brain slice preparations taken from morphine-dependent rats.[142,166] This lack of effect is in contrast to the strong withdrawal responses elicited by opiate antagonist injections directly into the locus coeruleus and suggests that the activation of this noradrenergic structure during morphine abstinence in the whole animal could be mediated by afferent neuronal projections to the locus coeruleus, which would be disrupted in brain slices. Several lines of evidence indicate that the projections responsible for the activation of the locus coeruleus during opiate withdrawal belong to those containing excitatory amino acids. The administration of antagonists of excitatory amino acid receptors into the lateral ventricle[167-169] or the locus coeruleus,[170] but not by peripheral route,[169] reduced the firing activation of locus coeruleus noradrenergic neurons induced by naloxone-precipitated withdrawal. A decrease in the severity of the somatic symptoms of morphine withdrawal was also observed after the administration of excitatory amino acid antagonists by the three different routes. In vivo voltammetric studies also found an attenuation of the hyperactivity induced in the locus coeruleus during naloxone-precipitated withdrawal by pretreatment with excitatory amino acid receptor antagonists in the lateral ventricle.[171] Accordingly, an increase in glutamate and aspartate efflux has been recently reported in the locus coeruleus during morphine withdrawal[172,173] that was directly correlated with the dose of naloxone used to precipitate withdrawal.[173] Little or no change was detected in immediate pericoerular locations, suggesting that such increases do not affect the immediate projection areas of the excitatory amino acid neurons activated under these conditions.[172] The afferent projections responsible for this effect seem to derive from the nucleus paragigantocellularis, one of the main excitatory amino acid inputs to the locus coeruleus since lesions of this area greatly attenuated withdrawal-induced activation of the locus coeruleus.[167]

However, more recent studies have reported a moderate increase in basal firing rates in locus coeruleus neurons in brain slices from opiate-dependent rats, which seems to be mediated by an upregulation of the intrinsic cAMP pathway.[174] The discrepancy with previous results may be explained, at least in part, by the relatively small number of cells tested in the other studies.[142,166] In addition, the increase in Fos-like immunoreactivity in the nucleus paragigantocellularis during opiate withdrawal was quite modest in comparison to the strong enhancement seen in locus coeruleus.[175,176] Besides, the administration of the hydrophilic opioid antagonist methylnaloxonium into the nucleus paragigantocellularis in morphine-dependent rats did not produce any relevant manifestation of withdrawal syndrome (Ruiz, Roques and Maldonado, unpublished observations). Taken together, these electrophysiological, biochemical and behavioral findings suggest that the withdrawal activation of the locus coeruleus is due both to cell bodies and/or nerve terminals that are supersensitive to the paragigantocellularis input.[175] Accordingly, recent studies found that chronic morphine administration to cultured noradrenergic neurons from the locus coeruleus caused an enhanced release of NA induced by various excitatory stimuli, including administration of excitatory amino acid, showing the existence of intrinsic adaptive changes of the locus coeruleus to chronic opiate exposure. This supersensitivity of locus coeruleus noradrenergic neurons was observed without opioid receptor desensitization and was probably due to changes in the postreceptor transduction system.[177]

Consequently, two different mechanisms seem to be responsible for the neuronal hyperactivity of the locus coeruleus during opiate withdrawal. First, an upregulation of the cAMP pathway occurs in the locus coeruleus that could induce several intrinsic modifications in this structure, such as a stimulation of neuronal physiological activity and an increase in the sensitivity to excitatory amino acid released from the afferents. The withdrawal effects observed after opiate antagonist administration into the locus coeruleus should be due to these intrinsic changes. The second mechanism would consist of an increased release of excitatory amino acids in the locus coeruleus, presumably due to the activation of neurons in the nucleus paragigantocellularis. In agreement with this hypothesis, firing rates in locus coeruleus neurons were double the control rates in brain slices,[174] whereas a 4-fold increase over control rates was reported during withdrawal in vivo.[149] This difference in the magnitude of the response is probably due to the effects induced in vivo by the second activator mechanism, i.e., the excitatory amino acid afferents from the paragigantocellularis.

PERIAQUEDUCTAL GRAY REGION

Various studies provide arguments to support the involvement of the periaqueductal gray matter in the expression of the physical component of opiate withdrawal. Thus, early studies show that the injections of opiate antagonists into the fourth ventricle were much more effective in precipitating abstinence in morphine-dependent animals than injections into the lateral and third ventricle.[178,179] Levallorphan also elicited a more severe degree of morphine abstinence when it was injected into the lower parts of the brain (midbrain and pontine levels).[179] Besides, the intracerebral application of crystalline naloxone in the diencephalic-mesencephalic juncture, near the periaqueductal gray matter, in opiate-dependent rats elicited a strong withdrawal syndrome.[123,180] However, taking into account the proximity of the site of injection to the ventricular space, the large amount of opiate antagonist administered (40-220 μg of crystalline naloxone) and the lipophilic properties of this antagonist, it cannot be excluded that some of the effects observed could be produced by a broad diffusion of the compound. When the hydrophilic opiate antagonist methylnaloxonium was locally administered into the periaqueductal gray matter at low doses (32-1000 ng), a severe withdrawal syndrome was also precipitated. The presence of some motor signs (rearing and hyperactivity) were particularly elevated.[181]

Another finding suggesting the involvement of the periaqueductal gray matter is the severe degree of physical dependence induced by the chronic local administration of opiates in this brain structure. Early studies already reported that the periaqueductal gray matter is very sensitive to developing dependence after local injection of enkephalin analogues[182] or morphine.[128] These results were recently confirmed by Bozarth.[160] In this study, morphine was chronically perfused into different brain structures related to opioid responses, and the maximal magnitude of physical dependence was induced by morphine infusions into the rostral part of the periaqueductal gray matter. The severity of naloxone-precipitated withdrawal was in this case comparable to that seen following repeated systemic administrations of morphine.[160]

The administration of protein kinase inhibitors into the periaqueductal gray matter was reported to strongly decrease the severity of naloxone-precipitated morphine withdrawal syndrome. This result suggests that such an intracellular signaling system plays an important role in the expression of dependence into the periaqueductal gray matter. As in the case of the locus coeruleus, kinases belonging to the serine/threonine kinase family seem to be selectively implicated. However, the reduced withdrawal response obtained in this structure was quantitatively less important than that observed after local administration into the locus coeruleus.[162] The local application of inhibitors of the enkephalin-degrading enzymes into the periaqueductal gray matter also blocked the expression of the naloxone-precipitated morphine withdrawal.[181] This decrease in the severity of abstinence was presumably induced by the increase of the opioid receptor occupation by endogenous peptides released into the periaqueductal gray matter and protected from their inactivation by the peptidase inhibitors. Therefore, during the morphine withdrawal a tonic- and/or naloxone-evoked release of enkephalins may occur in this brain structure.

The periaqueductal gray matter also plays an important role in other responses mediated by the opioid systems including analgesia,[183,184] but it does not seem to be implicated in the rewarding properties of opiates,[128] and it was not very sensitive to the methylnaloxonium-induced aversive stimulus of opiate abstinence.[130,131]

MESOLIMBIC SYSTEM

Several studies have identified the mesolimbic system (defined loosely as the ventral tegmental area, the mesolimbic dopamine system and the nucleus accumbens) as the most important substrate involved in several negative motivational aspects of opiate withdrawal. Indeed, the nucleus accumbens, one of the dopaminergic terminal regions in this system, has been reported to play a crucial role in the aversive stimulus properties of opiate withdrawal.[130,131] Very low doses of the opiate antagonist methylnaloxonium (4-64 ng) injected into the nucleus accumbens in morphine-dependent rats produced a disruption of food-motivated operant responding.[130] This nucleus was also the most sensitive structure to produce a place aversion, measured by using the place preference paradigm, in dependent rats after local administration of methylnaloxonium (250-500 ng).[131] Interestingly, the rewarding properties of the opiates and the aversive stimulus of withdrawal seem to be mediated by the same neuroanatomical substrate. Thus, the nucleus accumbens is also an important structure for the acute reinforcing effects of opiates in nondependent rats intravenously self-administering heroin. Injections of methylnaloxonium into the nucleus accumbens were effective in altering heroin self-administration at doses 8-10 times less than those required to produce the same effect when injected into the lateral ventricle.[185]

The studies evaluating the participation of the nucleus accumbens in the expression of the somatic symptoms of physical opiate abstinence reported results that suggest some interesting relationships between physical withdrawal and motivational withdrawal. A lack of correlation between the manifestation of the physical somatic signs of withdrawal and the development of place aversion or the disruption of operant behavior was observed when administering methylnaloxonium in morphine-dependent rats, suggesting the implication of a different neuroanatomical substrate in these two processes.[129-131] These somatic signs appeared when administering the opiate antagonist in several brain structures, but not in the nucleus accumbens. Accordingly, with this hypothesis, a dissociation between the negative motivational component of opiate withdrawal appearing after the administration of very low doses of naloxone and the physical somatic signs which appear only with higher doses of the opiate antagonist has been recently reported.[186] In this case, only the incidence of one sign of withdrawal, mastication, was significant.[129] In addition, morphine infusions into the nucleus accumbens failed to produce an important degree of physical dependence.[160]

In apparent contradiction with these results, recent studies related the dopaminergic neurons of the nucleus accumbens with the expression of physical opiate withdrawal. Thus, the activation of dopaminergic D_2, but not D_1, receptors within the nucleus accumbens reduced the severity of the naloxone-precipitated morphine withdrawal syndrome, whereas the blockade of accumbal D_2 receptors in morphine-dependent animals precipitated somatic withdrawal symptoms.[187] Accordingly, several dopaminergic antagonists, such as haloperidol[188] and the D_2 selective antagonist raclopride,[189] have been reported to exacerbate the morphine withdrawal response in guinea pigs. Consequently, although the nucleus accumbens is probably not a major site for the initiation of physical opiate abstinence, it is a major site for the motivational effects of opiate withdrawal. Thus, it seems to have an important role in regulating circuits that drive somatic and aversive responses of opiate withdrawal.

Other studies have focused on the participation of another dopaminergic terminal area in the mesolimbic system, the amygdaloid complex. One of the first signs of evidence of the involvement of this brain site was reported by Kerr and Pozuelo,[190] showing that the electrolytic lesion of the amygdala blocked jumping behavior in dependent rats but failed to alter other withdrawal signs. Other authors[191] did not find any modification in the expression of the spontaneous morphine abstinence after such electrolytic lesions, although in that study jumping behavior was not investigated. Amygdaloid kindling has been shown to strongly attenuate the severity of opiate withdrawal syndrome.[192] In agreement with the results of Kerr and Pozuelo, Calvino et al[124] observed a selective elicitation of jumping behavior after injection of naloxone (10 µg) in a small volume into the amygdala in morphine-dependent rats. Tremblay and Charton,[193] using the same dose of naloxone (10 µg), revealed that wet dog shakes and jumping appeared to be localized to this structure. In contrast, the administration of methylnaloxonium into the amygdala induced only a very mild morphine withdrawal syndrome, weaker than the one observed after injection into the lateral ventricle, in which jumping, wet dog shakes and other major signs of abstinence were absent even when the antagonist was administered at the highest dose

(1 μg).[129] These discrepancies may be related to the higher doses used and to the higher diffusion of naloxone, a lipophilic opiate antagonist. Accordingly, the chronic infusion of morphine into the amygdala did not produce an important degree of physical dependence.[160] Although the role of the amygdala in the expression of the somatic symptoms of opiate withdrawal is questioned, this structure plays an important role in negative motivational aspects of opiate withdrawal. Thus, microinjection of relatively low doses of methylnaloxonium (1-2 μg) into the amygdala produced a strong place aversion in morphine-dependent rats.[131]

The mesencephalic structures containing the dopaminergic cell bodies and other projecting areas such as the cortical structures do not seem to play a significant role in the opiate dependence processes. Thus, the electrolytic lesion of the septum, cingulum and cortical regions did not modify the expression of morphine withdrawal syndrome in rats.[191,194] When morphine was chronically perfused into the frontal cortex and the ventral tegmental area, the systemic administration of naloxone did not precipitate a relevant withdrawal syndrome, indicating the lack of development of physical opiate dependence.[160] Some withdrawal signs were observed when using unangled cannulae to perfuse morphine into the ventral tegmental area, but this effect seems to be a result of diffusion up to the periventricular gray region since angling the cannulae to avoid this structure virtually eliminated withdrawal behavior.[160] In agreement with this result, the local injection of methylnaloxonium in the ventral tegmental area failed to precipitate the somatic signs of withdrawal in rats made physically dependent by systemic administration of morphine.[131] This brain site was also less sensitive than other mesolimbic sites to methylnaloxonium-precipitated place aversion in morphine-dependent animals. Studies performed in the ventral tegmental area also supported the hypothesis that morphine physical dependence is mediated by different mechanisms than the rewarding effects of opiates: rats quickly learned to press a lever for microinjection of morphine into the ventral tegmental area, but challenge by a narcotic antagonist produced no signs of physical withdrawal.[128]

THALAMUS AND HYPOTHALAMUS

Early studies reported that the medial thalamus was one of the most sensitive structures to precipitate the withdrawal syndrome by the application of a large amount of crystalline naloxone (40-220 µg) in morphine-dependent rats.[123,180] The local injection of a naloxone solution into the thalamus also precipitated a severe abstinence with the presence of major signs of withdrawal such as jumping and wet dog shakes.[193] In contrast, when the hydrophilic opiate antagonist methylnaloxonium was administered in this structure, only a very mild withdrawal was observed in which major signs of abstinence were absent even when the antagonist was administered at the highest dose (1 µg).[129] These discrepancies may be related to the higher doses used in previous studies and to the higher diffusion of the lipophilic opiate antagonist naloxone. The very close localization of the site of injection in the medial thalamus from the ventricle space may favor a widespread diffusion of this lipophilic antagonist.

In agreement with this observation, other studies using different approaches suggest that the thalamus does not participate in the expression of physical withdrawal. Thus, the electrolytic lesion of the thalamus did not alter the manifestation of physical opiate abstinence in rats.[194] In addition, the perfusion with morphine into the thalamus has been reported to be unable to develop any relevant degree of physical dependence.[160]

The involvement of the hypothalamus in opiate dependence was suggested in early studies by Wei et al.[195] This brain structure is closely related to the regulation of body temperature. These authors proposed the hypothesis that the generation of an error signal in central thermoregulatory systems, controlled by the hypothalamus, may account for the appearance of some precipitated abstinence signs. Accordingly, an increased firing of hypothalamus neurons was reported during morphine abstinence,[196] and it was proposed that this area may mediate some of the "heat-producing" signs, such as wet dog shakes, observed in withdrawing rats.[197] Recent results obtained with the local administration of opiate antagonists seem to confirm this hypothesis. Indeed, the administration of methylnaloxonium into the anterior hypothalamus produced an elevated incidence of wet dog shake behavior in mor-

phine-dependent rats.[129] Another finding supporting the role of
the hypothalamus in opiate dependence was reported by Calvino
et al.[124] These authors showed that the lesion of the ventromedial
nuclei of the hypothalamus reduced the incidence of several signs
of opiate abstinence. However, this type of lesion also interrupts
the medial forebrain bundle, which sends noradrenergic projections
from the locus coeruleus to other brain regions. Results obtained
after the local chronic infusion of opiate agonists are in disagree-
ment with the previous findings since morphine perfusion into
hypothalamus did not develop any relevant degree of physical
dependence.[160]

OTHER BRAIN STRUCTURES

Several other brain sites have also been related to opiate dependence. Certain ventral midbrain structures have been suggested
to participate in the expression of morphine withdrawal.[198] Indeed,
naloxone administration into the substantia nigra in morphine-
dependent rats precipitated a withdrawal syndrome. However, the
doses used (1-10 μg of naloxone) were high in comparison to those
of methylnaloxonium (32-1000 ng) reported to precipitate opiate
withdrawal in other brain structures,[129] considering that methylnaloxonium is approximately 10 times less potent than naloxone
(Koob, Randolph and Chavkin, unpublished observations). Moreover, the severity of the withdrawal syndrome induced when
naloxone was administered into the substantia nigra at a moderate
dose (1 μg) was mild; only the presence of teeth chattering, hyperactivity and squealing was significantly elicited. Jumping, which is
a prominent withdrawal sign observed after central injection of
opiate antagonists,[129] was not reported after naloxone administration into the substantia nigra.[198] Furthermore, jumping and escape
attempts were not observed when injecting selective μ–, δ– or κ–
antagonists into this structure.[199]

The nucleus raphe magnus has also been reported to participate in the expression of withdrawal. Early studies show that the
lesion of the raphe nuclei blocked jumping behavior in dependent
rats but failed to alter other withdrawal signs.[200] A significant correlation between the hyperalgesia and the increased cellular activity has been recently observed during opiate abstinence in this

nucleus.[201] Furthermore, the injection of methylnaloxonium into the nucleus raphe magnus produced the presence of several somatic signs of opiate withdrawal in morphine-dependent rats. The incidence of wet dog shake behavior was particularly severe in this case.[129] The nucleus raphe magnus is one of the most prominent serotonergic structures that projects its fibers to various brain structures.[133] The activation of the serotonergic system has been reported to play an important role in the expression of wet dog shake behavior.[202] Shaking behavior is induced in nondependent rats by stimulation of the hippocampus,[203] but this structure does not seem to be related to wet dog shakes observed during the morphine withdrawal syndrome,[204] although other studies suggest that the hippocampus could be involved in some manifestations of morphine abstinence.[205] Wet dog shakes, as well as jumping behavior, were also reported to appear when administering a high dose of naloxone (10 µg in 0.1 µl) into the globus pallidus in opiate-dependent rats.[193] However, this effect does not seem to be specific to the globus pallidus and could be due to a diffusion of the elevated amount of naloxone administered. Accordingly, morphine perfusion into the proximity of the globus pallidus did not induce physical dependence.[160] Morphine perfusion into the reticular formation produced an appreciable degree of dependence, although this effect could result from drug diffusion to the periventricular gray region which was very close to the infusion site.[160]

Several studies have showed that the spinal cord is involved in the manifestation of several symptoms of opiate abstinence. Thus, the intrathecal administration of naloxone in morphine-dependent rats elicits a complete withdrawal syndrome characterized by behavioral and automonic symptoms.[155,206] The intrathecal route was the most sensitive to naloxone-induced jumping behavior in mice. The ED50 value obtained by this route was 10 and 25 times lower, respectively, than those obtained after the intracerebroventricular and subcutaneous administration.[207] In addition, the maximum frequency of jumping appeared 5 minutes after intrathecal naloxone, but it took more than 10 minutes to reach the most frequent jumping after subcutaneous and intracerebroventricular administration of naloxone.[207] Spinal sites are also important for the expression of other signs, such as diarrhea, which may reflect an abnormal function of the autonomic system.[208] However, a synergistic interaction between supraspinal and spinal sites seems to occur for the manifestation of these signs of withdrawal.[207,208] Some autonomic manifestations of abstinence, such as the increase in mean arterial pressure and heart rate, were also observed after intrathecal naloxone in spinal-transected dependent rats.[154,155] The surgical lesion of the afferent dorsal root fibers blocks withdrawal-associated hypertensive response, suggesting that input from peripheral systems to the spinal cord is involved in autonomic symptoms of withdrawal. Therefore, the spinal cord, interacting with cells of the preganglionic sympathetic neurons, seems to mediate the augmented sympathetic activity observed during withdrawal.[153,156] This hyperactivity of the sympathetic system is characterized in humans by several clinical manifestations of abstinence, such as mydriasis, perspiration, and respiratory and cardiovascular responses.[176]

REFERENCES

1. Koob GF, Bloom FE. Cellular and molecular mechanisms of drug dependence. Science 1988; 242:715-723.
2. Koob GF, Stinus L, Le Moal M et al. Opponent process theory of motivation: Neurobiological evidence from studies of opiate dependence. Neurosci Biobehav Rev 1989; 13:135-140.
3. Solomon RL. The opponent process theory of acquired motivation. Am Psychol 1980; 35:691-712.
4. Solomon RL. Acquired motivation and affective opponent processes. In: Madden IV, ed. Neurobiology of Learning, Emotion and Affect. NY: Raven Press, Ltd., 1991:307-347.
5. Collier HOJ. A general theory of the genesis of drug dependence by induction of receptors. Nature 1965; 205:181-183.
6. Chang KJ, Eckel RW, Blanchard SG. Opioid peptides induced reduction of enkephalin receptors in cultured neuroblastoma cells. Nature 1982; 296:446-448.
7. Law PY, Hom DS, Loh HH. Downregulation of opiate receptor in neuroblastoma x glioma NG 10815 hybrid cells. J Biol Chem 1984; 259:4096-4104.
8. Puttfarcken PS, Cox BM. Morphine-induced desensitization and downregulation at mu-receptor in 7315C pituitary tumor cells. Life Sci 1989; 45:1937-1942.
9. Zadina JE, Kastin AJ, Kersh D et al. TYR-MIF and hemorphin can act as opiate agonist as well as antagonist in the guinea pig ileum. Life Sci 1992; 51:869-885.

10. Morris BJ, Herz A. Control of opiate receptor number in vivo: Simultaneous kappa-receptor downregulation and mu-receptor upregulation following chronic agonist/antagonist treatment. Neuroscience 1989; 29:433-442.

11. Rothman RB. A review of the role of anti-opioid peptides in morphine tolerance and dependence. Synapse 1992; 12:129-138.

12. Werling LL, McMahon PN, Cox BM. Selective changes in mu-opioid receptor properties induced by chronic morphine exposure. Proc Natl Acad Sci USA 1989; 86:6393-6397.

13. Yoburn BC, Duttaroy A, Billings B. Dose-dependent downregulation of opioid receptors in mice. Keystone, Colorado: Abstracts, INRC, 1992.

14. Nestler EJ. Molecular mechanisms of drug addiction. J Neurosci 1992; 12:2439-2450.

15. Terwilliger RZ, Beitner-Johnson D, Sevatino KA et al. A general role for adaptations in G-proteins and the cyclic AMP system in mediating the chronic actions of morphine and cocaine on neuronal function. Brain Res 1991; 548:100-110.

16. Bronstein DM, Przewlocki R, Akil H. Effects of morphine treatment on pro-opio-melanocortin systems in rat brain. Brain Res 1990; 519:102-111.

17. Hammonds RG, Nicholas P, Li CH. Beta-endorphin (1-27) is an antagonist of beta-endorphin analgesia. Proc Natl Acad Sci USA 1984; 81:1389-1393.

18. Nicolas P, Hammonds RG, Li CH. Beta-endorphin analgesia is inhibited by synthetic analogs of beta-endorphin. Proc Natl Acad Sci USA 1984; 81:3074-3077.

19. Schulteis G, Markou A, Gold L et al. Relative sensitivity to naloxone of multiple indices of opiate withdrawal: A quantitative dose-response analysis. J Pharmacol Exp Ther 1994; 271:1391-1398.

20. Wei EL, Loh HH, Way EL. Quantitative aspects of abstinence in morphine-dependent rats. J Pharmacol Exp Ther 1973; 184:398-403.

21. Faris PK, Komisaruk BR, Watkins LR et al. Evidence for the neuropeptide cholecystokinin as an antagonist of opiate analgesia. Science 1983; 219:310-312.

22. Galina ZH, Kastin AJ. Existence of antiopiate systems as illustrated by MIF-1/Tyr-MIF-1. Life Sci 1986; 39:2153-2159.

23. Yang HYT, Fratta W, Majane EA et al. Isolation sequencing, synthesis and pharmacological characterization of two brain neuropeptides that modulate the action of morphine. Proc Natl Acad Sci USA 1985; 82:7757-7761.

24. Rehfeld JL. Neuronal cholecystokinin. One or two multiple transmitters. J Neurochem 1985; 44:1-10.

25. Gibbs J, Young RC, Smith GP. Cholecystokinin elicits satiety in rats with open gatric fistulas. Nature 1973; 245:323-325.

26. Daugé V, Steimes P, Derrien M et al. CCK-8 effects on motivational and emotional states of rats involve CCK-A receptors of the posteromedial part of the nucleus accumbens. Pharmacol Biochem Behav 1989; 34:157-163.

27. Innis RB, Snyder SH. Cholecystokinin receptor binding in brain and pancreas. Regulation of pancreatic binding by cyclic and acyclic guanine nucleotides. Eur J Pharmacol 1980; 65:123-124.

28. Moran TH, Robinson PH, Goldrich MS et al. Two brain cholecystokinin receptors: Implication for behavioral actions. Brain Res 1986; 362:175-179.

29. Durieux C, Ruiz-Gayo M, Roques BP. In vivo binding affinities of cholecystokinin agonists and antagonists determined using the selective CCK-B agonist [^{3}H]pBC 264. Eur J Pharmacol 1991; 209:185-193.

30. Kopin AS, Lee YM, McBride EW et al. Expression cloning and characterization of the canine parietal cell gastrin receptor. Proc Natl Acad Sci USA 1992; 89:3605-3609.

31. Wank SA, Harkins R, Jensen RT et al. Purification, molecular cloning and functional expression of the cholecystokinin receptor from rat pancreas. Proc Natl Acad Sci USA 1992; 89:3125-3129.

32. Lee YM, Beinborn M, McBride EW et al. The human brain cholecystokinin-B/gastrin receptor. J Biol Chem 1993; 268:8164-8169.

33. Hill DR, Woodruff GN. Differentiation of central cholecystokinin receptor binding sites using the non-peptide antagonists MK-329 and L-365,260. Brain Res 1990; 526:276-283.

34. Faris PK. Opiate antagonist function of cholecystokinin in analgesia and energy balance systems. Ann NY Acad Sci 1985; 448:437-447.

35. Zetler G. Analgesia and ptosis caused by caerulein and cholecystokinin octapeptide (CCK-8). Neuropharmacology 1980; 19:415-422.

36. Baber NS, Dourish CT, Hill DR. The role of CCK, caerulein, and CCK antagonists in nociception. Pain 1989; 39:307-328.

37. Dourish CT, O'Neill MF, Couglan J et al. The selective CCK-B receptor antagonist L-365,260 enhances morphine analgesia and prevents morphine tolerance in the rat. Eur J Pharmacol 1990; 176:35-44.

38. Dourish CT, O'Neill MF, Schaeffer LW et al. The cholecystokinin receptor antagonist devazepide enhances morphine-induced analgesia but not morphine-induced respiratory depression in the squirrel monkey. J Pharmacol Exp Ther 1990; 255:1158-1165.

39. Lavigne GJ, Millington WR, Mueller GP. The CCK-A and CCK-B receptor antagonists, devazepide and L-365,260, enhance morphine

antinociception only in non-acclimated rats exposed to a novel environment. Neuropeptides 1992; 21:119-129.

40. Zhou Y, Sun YH, Zhang ZW et al. Increased release of immunoreactive cholecystokinin octapeptide by morphine and potentiation of mu-opioid analgesia by CCJ$_B$ receptor antagonist L-365,260 in rat spinal cord. Eur J Pharmacol 1993; 234:147-154.

41. Maldonado R, Derrien M, Noble F et al. Association of the peptidase inhibitor RB 101 and a CCK-B antagonist strongly enhances antinociceptive responses. NeuroReport 1993; 7:947-950.

42. Valverde O, Maldonado R, Fournié-Zaluski MC et al. CCK-B antagonists strongly potentiate antinociception mediated by endogenous enkephalins. J Pharmacol Exp Ther 1994; 270:77-88.

43. Valverde O, Blommaert A, Turcaud S et al. The CCK-B antagonist PD-134,308 induces a long-lasting potentiation of antinociceptive responses mediated by endogenous enkaphalins in the rat tail-flick test. Eur J Pharmacol 1995; 286:79-93.

44. Rattray M, Jordan CC, De Belleroche J. The novel CCK antagonist L-364,718 abolished caerulein- but potentiated morphine-induced antinociception. Eur J Pharmacol 1988; 152:163-166.

45. O'Neill MF, Dourish CT, Iversen SD. Morphine analgesia in the rat paw pressure test is blocked by CCK and enhanced by the CCK antagonist MK-329. Neuropharmacology 1989; 28:243-248.

46. Suh HH, Tseng LF. Differential effects of sulfated cholecystokinin octapeptide and proglumide injected intrathecally on antinociception induced by beta-endorphin and morphine administered intracerebroventricularly in mice. Eur J Pharmacol 1990; 179:329-339.

47. Wiesenfeld-Hallin Z, Xu XJ, Hughes J et al. PD-134,308, a selective antagonist of cholecystokinin type B receptor, enhances the analgesic effect of morphine and synergistically interacts with intrathecal galanin to depress spinal nociceptive reflexes. Proc Natl Acad Sci USA 1990; 87:7105-7109.

48. Kellstein DE, Price DD, Mayer DE. Cholecystokinin and its antagonist lorgumide respectively attenuate and facilitate morphine-induced inhibition of C-fiber evoked discharges of dorsal horn nociceptive neurons. Brain Res 1991; 540:302-306.

49. Sullivan AF, Hewett K, Dickenson AH. Differential modulation of alpha 2-adrenergic and opioid spinal antinociception by cholecystokinin and cholecystokinin antagonists in the rat dorsal horn: An electrophysiological study. Brain Res 1994; 662:141-147.

50. Stengaard-Pedersen K, Larson LI. Localization and opiate receptor binding of enkephalin, CCK and ACTH/beta-endorphin in the rat central nervous system. Peptides 1981; 2:3-19.

51. Xu XJ, Puke MJC, Verge VMK et al. Upregulation of cholecystokinin in primary sensory neurons is associated with morphine in-

sensitivity in experimental neuropathic pain in rat. Neurosci Lett 1993; 152:129-132.

52. Kapas L, Benedek G, Penek B. Cholecystokinin interferes with the thermoregulatory effects of exogenous and endogenous opioids. Neuropeptides 1989; 14:85-92.

53. Ben-Horin N, Ben-Horin E, Frenk H. The effects of proglumide on morphine-induced mortility changes. Psychopharmacology 1984; 84:541-543.

54. Schnur P, Raigoza VP, Sanchez MR et al. Cholecystokinin antagonizes morphine-induced hypoactivity and hyperactivity in hamsters. Pharmacol Biochem Behav 1986; 25:1067-1070.

55. Schnur P, Cesar SS, Foderaro MA et al. Efffects of cholecystokinin on morphine-elicited hyperactivity in hamsters. Pharmacol Biochem Behav 1991; 39:581-586.

56. Miller KK, Lupica CR. Morphine-induced excitation of pyramidal neurons is inhibited by cholecystokinin in the CA1 region of the rat hippocampal slice. J Pharmacol Exp Ther 1994; 268:753-761.

57. Itoh S, Katsuura G. Effects of beta-endorphin, thyrotropin-releasing hormone and cholecystokinin on body-shaking behavior in rats. Jpn J Physiol 1982; 32:667-675.

58. Higgins GA, Nguyen P, Sellers EM. Morphine place conditioning is differentially affected by CCK-A and CCK-B receptor antagonists. Brain Res 1992; 572:208-215.

59. Harro J, Vasar E, Bradwejn J. CCK in animal and human research on anxiety. TIPS 1993; 14:244-249.

60. Smadja C, Maldonado R, Turcaud S et al. Opposite role of CCK-A and CCK-B receptors in the modulation of endogenous enkephalins' antidepressant-like effects. Psychopharmacology 1995; 120:400-408.

61. Noble F, Smadja C, Roques BP. Role of endogenous cholecystokinin in the facilitation of mu-mediated antinociception by delta opioid agonists. J Pharmacol Exp Ther 1994; 271:1127-1134.

62. Faris PK, Beinfeld MC, Scallet AC et al. Increase in hypothalamic cholecystokinin following acute and chronic morphine. Brain Res 1986; 367:405-407.

63. Benoleil JJ, Bourgoin S, Mauborgne A et al. Differential inhibitory/stimulatory modulation of spinal CCK release by mu-opioid and delta-opioid agonists, and selective blockade of mu-dependent inhibition by k receptor stimulation. Neurosci Lett 1991; 124:204-207.

64. Benoleil JJ, Mauborgne A, Bourgoin S et al. Opioid control of the in vivo release of CCK-like material from the rat substantia nigra. J Neurochem 1992; 58:916-920.

65. Rattray M, De Belleroche J. Morphine action on cholecystokinin

octapeptide release from rat periaqueductal gray slices: Sensitization by naloxone. Neuropeptides 1987; 10:189-200.

66. Rodriguez RE, Sacristan MP. In vivo release of CCK-8 from the dorsal horn of the rat: Inhibition by DAGOL. FEBS Lett 1989; 250:215-217.

67. Ruiz-Gayo M, Durieux C, Fournié-Zaluski MC et al. Stimulation of delta opioid receptors reduces the in vivo binding of the CCK-B-selective agonist [^{3}H]pBC 264: Evidence for a physiological regulation of CCKergic systems by endogenous enkephalins. J Neurochem 1992; 59:1805-1811.

68. Gall C, Lauterborn J, Burks D et al. Co-localization of enkephalins and cholecystokinin in discrete areas of rat brain. Brain Res 1987; 403:403-408.

69. Pohl M, Benoliel JJ, Bourgoin S et al. Regional distribution of calcitonin gene-related peptide-, substance P-, cholecystokinin-, Met^5-enkephalin-, and dynorphin A (1-8)-like materials in the spinal cord and dorsal root ganglia of adult rats: Effects of dorsal rhizotomy and neonatal capsaicin. J Neurochem 1990; 55: 1122-1130.

70. Tang J, Chou J, Iadarola M et al. Proglumide prevents and curtails acute tolerance to morphine in rats. Neuropharmacology 1984; 23:715-718.

71. Watkins LR, Kinscheck IB, Mayer DJ. Potentiation of morphine analgesia and apparent reversal of morphine tolerance by proglumide. Science 1984; 224:395-396.

72. Panerai AE, Rovati LC, Cocco E et al. Dissociation of tolerance and dependence to morphine: A possible role for cholecystokinin. Brain Res 1987; 410:52-60.

73. Dourish CT, Hawley D, Iversen SD. Enhancement of morphine analgesia and prevention of morphine tolerance in the rat by the cholecystokinin antagonist L-364,718. Eur J Pharmacol 1988; 147:469-472.

74. Ding XZ, Fan SG, Han JS. Reversal of tolerance to morphine but no potentiation of morphine-induced analgesia by antiserum against cholecystokinin octapeptide. Neuropharmacology 1986; 25: 1155-1160.

75. Xu XJ, Wiesenfeld-Hallin Z, Hughes J et al. CI988, a selective antagonist of cholecystokinin-B receptors, prevents morphine tolerance in rats. Br J Pharmacol 1992; 105:591-596.

76. Ding XZ, Bayer BM. Increases of CCK mRNA and peptide in different brain areas following acute and chronic administration of morphine. Brain Res 1993; 625:139-144.

77. Pu S, Zhuang H, Lu Z et al. Cholecystokinin gene expression in rat amygdaloid neurons: Normal distribution and effect of morphine tolerance. Mol Brain Res 1994; 21:183-189.

78. Maldonado R, Valverde O, Ducos B et al. Inhibition of morphine withdrawal syndrome by the association of a peptidase inhibitor and a CCK-B antagonist. Br J Pharmacol 1995; 114:1031-1039.

79. Hughes J, Boden P, Costall B et al. Development of a class of selective cholecystokinin type B receptor antagonists having potent anxiolytic activity. Proc Natl Acad Sci USA 1990; 87:6728-6732.

80. Pournaghash S, Riley A. Failure of cholecystokinin to precipitate withdrawal in morphine-treated rats. Pharmacol Biochem Behav 1991; 38:479-484.

81. Maldonado R, Valverde O, Derrien M et al. Effects induced by BC 264, a selective agonist of CCK-B receptors, on morphine-dependent rats. Pharmacol Biochem Behav 1994; 48:363-369.

82. Charpentier B, Durieux C, Pélaprat D et al. Enzyme-resistant CCK analogs with high affinities for central receptors. Peptides 1988; 9:835-841.

83. Derrien M, Noble F, Maldonado R et al. CCK-A or CCK-B receptor activation leads to antinociception or to hyperalgesia, respectively: Evidence for an indirect interaction with the opioidergic system. Neurosci Lett 1993; 160:193-196.

84. Koob GF, Maldonado R, Stinus L. Neural substrates of opiate withdrawal. Trends Neurosci 1992; 15:186-191.

85. Ravard S, Dourish T. Cholecystokinin and anxiety. Trends Pharmacol Sci 1990; 11:271-273.

86. Costall B, Domeney AM, Hughes J et al. Anxiolytic effects of CCK-B antagonists. Neuropeptides 1991; 19(Suppl):65-73.

87. Dockray GJ, Vaillant C, Williams RG. New vertebrate brain-gut peptide related to a molluscan neuropeptide and an opioid peptide. Nature 1981; 293:656-657.

88. Weber E, Evans CJ, Samuelsson SJ et al. Novel peptide neuronal system in rat brain and pituitary. Science 1981; 214:1248-1251.

89. Allard M, Theodosis DT, Rousselot P et al. Characterization and localization of a putative morphine-modulating peptide, FLFQPQRFamide, in the rat spinal cord: Biochemical and immunocytochemical studies. Neuroscience 1991; 40:81-92.

90. Kivipelto L, Majane EA, Yang HY et al. Immunohistochemical distribution and partial characterization of FLFQPQRFamide-like peptides in the central nervous system. J Comp Neurol 1989; 286:269-287.

91. Kivipelto L, Panula P. Origin and distribution of neuropeptide-FF-like immunoreactivity in the spinal cord of rats. J Comp Neurol 1991; 307:107-119.

92. Majane EA, Panula P, Yang HY. Rat brain regional distribution and spinal cord neuronal pathway of FLFQPQRF-NH2, a mammalian FMRF-NH2-like peptide. Brain Res 1989; 494:1-12.

93. Allard M, Geoffre S, Legendre P et al. Characterization of rat spinal cord receptors to FLFQPQRFamide, a mammalian morphine modulating peptide: A binding study. Brain Res 1989; 500:169-176.

94. Allard M, Zajac JM, Simonnet G. Autoradiographic distribution of receptors to FLFQPQRFamide, a morphine-modulating peptide, in the rat central nervous system. Neuroscience 1992; 49:101-116.

95. Kavaliers M, Hirst M. FMRFamide, a putative endogenous opiate antagonist: Evidence from suppression of defeat-induced analgesia and feeding in mice. Neuropeptides 1985; 6:485-494.

96. Kavaliers M, Hirst M. Inhibitory influences of FMRFamide and PLG on stress-induced opioid analgesia and activity. Brain Res 1986; 372:370-374.

97. Kavaliers M. Inhibitory influences of mammalian FMRFamide (Phe-Met-Arg-Phe-amide)-related peptides on nociception and morphine- and stress-induced analgesia in mice. Neurosci Lett 1990; 115:307-312.

98. Oberling P, Stinus L, Le Moal M et al. Biphasic effect on nociception and antiopiate activity of the neuropeptide FF (FLFQPQRFamide) in the rat. Peptides 1993; 14:919-924.

99. Kavaliers M, Hirst M, Mathers A. Inhibitory influences of FMRF amide on morphine- and deprivation-induced feeding. Neuroendocrinology 1985; 40:533-535.

100. Kavaliers M, Yang HYT. IgG from antiserum against endogenous mammalian FMRF-NH2-related peptides augments morphine- and stress-induced analgesia in mice. Peptides 1989; 10:741-745.

101. Lake JR, Hammond MV, Shaddox RC et al. IgG from neuropeptide FF antiserum reverses morphine tolerance in the rat. Neurosci Lett 1991; 132:29-32.

102. Lake JR, Hebert KM, Payza K et al. Analog of neuropeptide FF attenuates morphine tolerance. Neurosci Lett 1992; 146:203-206.

103. Tang J, Yang HY, Costa E. Inhibition of spontaneous and opiate-modified nociception by an endogenous neuropeptide with Phe-Met-Arg-Phe-NH2-like immunoreactivity. Proc Natl Acad Sci USA 1984; 81:5002-5005.

104. Rothman RB, Brady LS, Xu H et al. Chronic intracerebroventricular infusion of the antiopioid peptide, Phe-Leu-Phe-Gln-Pro-Gln-ArgPhe-NH2 (NPFF), downregulates mu opioid binding sites in rat brain. Peptides 1993; 14:1271-1277.

105. Magnuson DSK, Sullivan AF, Simonnet G et al. Differential interaction of cholecystokinin and FLFQPQRF-NH2 with mu and delta opioid antinociception in the rat spinal cord. Neuropeptides 1990; 16:213-218.

106. Malin DH, Lake JR, Fowler DE et al. FMRF-NH2-like mammalian peptide precipitates opiate-withdrawal syndrome in the rat. Peptides 1990; 11:277-280.

107. Malin DH, Lake JR, Hammond MV et al. FMRF-NH2-like mammalian octapeptide: Possible role in opiate dependence and abstinence. Peptides 1990; 11:969-972.

108. Malin DH, Lake JR, Leyva JE et al. Analog of neuropeptide FF attenuates morphine abstinence syndrome. Peptides 1991; 12:1011-1014.

109. Stinus L, Allard M, Gold L et al. Changes in CNS neuropeptide FF-like material, pain sensitivity, and opiate dependence following chronic morphine treatment. Peptides 1995; 16:1235-1241.

110. Trujillo KE, Akil H. Inhibition of morphine tolerance and dependence by the NMDA receptor antagonist MK-801. Science 1991; 251:85-87.

111. Devillers JP, Simonnet G. Modulation of neuropeptide FF release from rat spinal cord slices by glutamate. Involvement of NMDA receptors. Eur J Pharmacol 1994; 271:185-192.

112. Hoffman O, Wiesenfeld-Hallin Z. The CCK-B receptor antagonist CI988 reverses tolerance to morphine in rats. NeuroReport 1994; 5:2565-2568.

113. Corbett AD, Paterson SJ, McKnight AT et al. Dynorphin are ligands for the kappa-subtype of opiate receptor. Nature 1982; 299:79-81.

114. Friedman HJ, Jen MF, Chang JK et al. Dynorphin: A possible modulatory peptide on morphine or beta-endorphin analgesia in mice. Eur J Pharmacol 1981; 69:357-360.

115. Fujimoto J, Arts KS. Clonidine, administered intracerebroventricularly in mice, produces an antianalgesic effect which may be mediated spinally by dynorphin A(1-17). Neuropharmacology 1990; 29:351-358.

116. Fujimoto J, Arts KS, Rady J et al. Spinal dynorphin A(1-17): Possible mediator of antianalgesic action. Neuropharmacology 1990; 29:609-617.

117. Fujimoto J, Arts KS, Rady J et al. Intracerebroventricular analgesia enhanced by intrathecal dynorphin A(1-17) antibody. Prog Clin Biol 1990; 328:433-436.

118. Fujimoto J, Holmes B. Systemic single-dose morphine pretreatment desensitizes mice to the spinal antianalgesic action of dynorphin A(1-17). J Pharmacol Exp Ther 1990; 254:1-7.

119. Jones DNC, Holtzman SG. Long-term kappa-opioid receptor blockade following nor-binaltorphimine. Eur J Pharmacol 1992; 215:345-348.

120. Spanagel R, Almeida OFX, Bartl C et al. Endogenous kappa-opioid systems in opiate withdrawal: Role in aversion and accompanying changes in mesolimbic dopamine release. Psychopharmacology 1994; 115:121-127.

121. Maldonado R, Negus S, Koob GF. Precipitation of morphine withdrawal syndrome in rats by administration of mu-, delta- and kappa-selective opioid antagonists. Neuropharmacology 1992; 31: 1231-1241.

122. Suzuki T, Narita M, Takahahi Y et al. Effects of nor-binaltorphimine on the development of analgesic tolerance to and physical dependence on morphine. Eur J Pharmacol 1992; 213:91-97.

123. Wei E, Loh HH, Way EL. Brain sites of precipitated abstinence in morphine-dependent rats. J Pharmacol Exp Ther 1973; 185: 108-115.

124. Calvino B, Lagowska J, Ben-Ari Y. Morphine withdrawal syndrome: Differential participation of structures located within the amygdaloid complex and striatum of the rat. Brain Res 1979; 177:19-34.

125. Routtenberg A, Sladek J, Bondareff W. Historical fluorescence after application of neurochemicals to caudate nucleus and septal area in vivo. Science 1968; 161:272-274.

126. Bondareff W, Routtenberg A, Narotzky R et al. Intrastriatal spreading of biogenic amines. Exp Neurol 1970; 28:213-229.

127. Schroeder RL, Weinger MB, Vakassian L et al. Methylnaloxonium diffuses out of the brain more slowly than naloxone after direct intracerebral injection. Neurosci Lett 1991; 121:173-177.

128. Bozarth MA, Wise RA. Anatomically distinct opiate receptor fields mediate reward and physical dependence. Science 1984; 224: 516-517.

129. Maldonado R, Stinus L, Gold LH et al. Role of different brain structures in the expression of the physical morphine withdrawal syndrome. J Pharmacol Exp Ther 1992; 261:669-677.

130. Koob GF, Wall TL, Bloom FE. Nucleus accumbens as a substrate for the aversive stimulus effects of opiate withdrawal. Psychopharmacology (Berlin) 1989; 98:530-534.

131. Stinus L, Le Moal M, Koob GF. The nucleus accumbens and amygdala as possible substrates for the aversive stimulus effects of opiate withdrawal. Neuroscience 1990; 37:767-773.

132. Maldonado R, Koob GF. Modification in the development of morphine dependence in rats by electrolytic lesion of the locus coeruleus. Brain Res 1993; 605:128-138.

133. Dahlström A, Fuxe K. Evidence for the existence of monoamine-containing neurons in the central nervous system. I. Demonstration of monoamines in the cell bodies of brain stem neurons. Acta Physiol Scand 1965; 232(Suppl):1-55.

134. Foote SL, Bloom FE, Aston-Jones G. Nucleus locus ceruleus: New evidence of anatomical and physiological specificity. Physiol Rev 1983; 63:844-914.

135. Moore RY, Bloom FE. Central catecholamine neuron systems:

Anatomy and physiology of the norepinephrine and epinephrine systems. Annu Rev Neurosci 1979; 2:113-168.

136. Aghajanian GG, Wang YY. Common alpha-2 and opiate effector mechanisms in the locus coeruleus intracellular studies in brain slices. Neuropharmacology 1987; 26:793-799.

137. Redmond DE, Jr., Huang YH, Snyder DR et al. Behavioral effects of stimulation of the nucleus locus coeruleus in the stump-tailed monkey (Maccaca arctoides). Brain Res 1976; 116:502-510.

138. Redmond DE Jr, Huang YH. Current concepts II. New evidence for a locus coeruleus-norepinephrine connection with anxiety. Life Sci 1979; 25:2149-2162.

139. Redmond DE Jr, Huang YH. The primate locus coeruleus and effects of clonidine on opiate withdrawal. J Clin Psychiatry 1982; 46:25-29.

140. Grant SJ, Huang YH, Redmond E Jr. Behavior of monkeys during opiate withdrawal and locus coeruleus stimulation. Pharmacol Biochem Behav 1988; 30:13-19.

141. Bird SJ, Kuhar MJ. Iontophoretic application of opiates to the locus coeruleus. Brain Res 1977; 122:523-533.

142. Andrade R, Vandermaelen CP, Aghajanian GK. Morphine tolerance and dependence in the locus coeruleus: Single-cell studies in brain slices. Eur J Pharmacol 1983; 91:161-169.

143. Aghajanian GK. Tolerance of locus coeruleus neurons to morphine and suppression of withdrawal response by clonidine. Nature 1978; 276:186-188.

144. Llorens C, Martres M, Bardry M et al. Hypersensitivity to noradrenaline in cortex after chronic morphine: Relevance to tolerance and dependence. Nature 1978; 274:603-605.

145. Laverty R, Roth RH. Clonidine reverses the increased norepinephrine turnover during morphine withdrawal in rats. Brain Res 1980; 182:482-485.

146. Crawley JN, Laverty R, Roth RH. Clonidine reversal of increased norepinephrine metabolite levels during morphine withdrawal. Eur J Pharmacol 1979; 57:247-250.

147. DiStefano PS, Brown OM. Biochemical correlates of morphine withdrawal. 2. Effects of clonidine. J Pharmacol Exp Ther 1985; 233:339-344.

148. Nestler EJ, Tallman JF. Chronic morphine treatment increases cyclic AMP-dependent protein kinase activity in the rat locus coeruleus. Mol Pharmacol 1988; 33:127-132.

149. Rasmussen K, Beitner-Johnson DB, Krystal JH et al. Opiate withdrawal and rat locus coeruleus: Behavioral, electrophysiological, and biochemical correlates. J Neurosci 1990; 10:2308-2317.

150. Esposito E, Kruszewska A, Ossowska G et al. Noradrenergic and

behavioral effects of naloxone injected into the locus coeruleus of morphine-dependent rats and their control by clonidine. Psychopharmacology 1987; 93:393-396.

151. Glick SD, Charap AD. Morphine dependence in rats with medial forebrain bundle lesions. Psychopharmacologia (Berlin) 1973; 34:343-348.

152. Britton KT, Svensson T, Schwartz J et al. Dorsal noradrenergic bundle lesions fail to alter opiate withdrawal or suppression of opiate withdrawal by clonidine. Life Sci 1984; 34:133-139.

153. Franz DN, Hare BD, McCloskey KL. Spinal sympathetic neurons: Possible sites of opiate withdrawal suppression by clonidine. Science 1982; 215:1643-1645.

154. Delander,GE, Takemori AE. Spinal antagonism of tolerance and dependence induced by systemically administered morphine. Eur J Pharmacol 1983; 94:35-42.

155. Turner RM, Marshall DC, Buccafusco JJ. Supraspinal and spinal components of naloxone-induced morphine withdrawal. Pharmacologist 1984; 26:197.

156. Buccafusco JJ, Marshall DC. Dorsal root lesions block the expression of morphine withdrawal elicited from the rat spinal cord. Neurosci Lett 1985; 59:319-324.

157. Friedler G, Bhargava HN, Quock R et al. The effect of 6-hydroxydopamine on morphine tolerance and physical dependence. J Pharmacol Exp Ther 1972; 183:49-55.

158. Elchisak MA, Rosecrans JA. Development of morphine tolerance and physical dependence in rats depleted of brain catecholamines by 6-hydroxydopamine. Neuropharmacology 1979; 18:175-182.

159. Funada M, Suzuki T, Sugano Y et al. Role of the β-adrenoceptors in the expression of morphine withdrawal signs. Life Sci 1994; 54:113-118.

160. Bozarth MA. Physical dependence produced by central morphine infusions: An anatomical mapping study. Neurosci Biobehav Rev 1994; 18:373-383.

161. Matsuoka I, Maldonado R, Defer N et al. Chronic morphine administration causes region-specific increase of brain type VIII adenylyl cyclase mRNA. Eur J Pharmacol Mol Sect 1994; 268:215-221.

162. Maldonado R, Valverde O, Garbay C et al. Protein kinases mediate the expression of opiate withdrawal in the locus coeruleus and periaqueductal gray matter. Naunyn Schmiedebergs Arch Pharmacol 1995; 352:565-575.

163. Maldonado R, Feger J, Fournié-Zaluski MC et al. Differences in physical dependence induced by selective mu or delta opioid agonists and by endogenous enkephalins protected by peptidase inhibitors. Brain Res 1990; 520:247-254.

164. Noble F, Coric P, Fournié-Zaluski MC et al. Lack of physical dependence in mice after repeated systemic administration of the mixed inhibitor prodrug of enkephalin-degrading enzymes RB 101. Eur J Pharmacol 1992; 223:91-96.

165. Williams JT, Christie MJ, North RA et al. Potentiation of enkephalin action by peptidase inhibitors in rat locus coeruleus in vitro. J Pharmacol Exp Ther 1987; 243:397-401.

166. Christie MJ, Williams JT, North RA. Cellular mechanisms of opioid tolerance: Studies in single brain neurons. J Pharmacol Exp Ther 1987; 32:633-638.

167. Rasmussen K, Aghajanian GK. Withdrawal-induced activation of locus coeruleus neurons in opiate-dependent rats: Attenuation by lesion of the nucleus paragigantocellularis. Brain Res 1989; 505:346-350.

168. Tung CS, Grenhoff J, Svensson TH. Morphine withdrawal responses of rat locus coeruleus neurons are blocked by an excitatory amino acid antagonist. Acta Physiol Scand 1990; 138:581-582.

169. Rasmussen K, Krystal JH, Aghajanian GK. Excitatory amino acids and morphine withdrawal: Differential effects of central and peripheral kynurenic acid administration. Psychopharmacology 1991; 105:508-512.

170. Akaoka A, Aston-Jones G. Opiate withdrawal-induced hyperactivity of locus coeruleus neurons is substantially mediated by augmented excitatory amino acid input. J Neurosci 1991; 11: 3830-3839.

171. Hong M, Milne B, Jhamandas K. Evidence for the involvement of excitatory amino acid pathways in the development of precipitated withdrawal from acute and chronic morphine: An in vivo voltammetric study in the rat locus coeruleus. Brain Res 1994; 623:131-141.

172. Aghajanian GK, Kogan JH, Moghaddam B. Opiate withdrawal increases glutamate and aspartate efflux in the locus coeruleus: An in vivo microdialysis study. Brain Res 1994; 636:126-130.

173. Zhang T, Feng Y, Rockhold RW et al. Naloxone-precipitated morphine withdrawal increases pontine glutamate levels in the rat. Life Sci 1994; 55:PL25-31.

174. Kogan JH, Nestler EJ, Aghajanian GK. Elevated basal firing rates and enhanced responses to 8-Br-cAMP in locus coeruleus nerons in brain slices from opiate-dependent rats. Eur J Pharmacol 1992; 211:47-53.

175. Hayward MD, Duman RS, Nestler EJ. Induction of the c-fos proto-oncogene during opiate withdrawal in the locus coeruleus and other regions of rat brain. Brain Res 1990; 525:256-266.

176. Stornetta RL, Norton FE, Guyenet PG. Autonomic areas of rat brain exhibit increased Fos-like immunoreactivity during opiate withdrawal in rats. Brain Res 1993; 624:19-28.
177. Ronken E, Mulder AH, Schoffelmeer ANM. Chronic activation of mu- and kappa-opioid receptors in cultured catecholaminergic neurons from rat brain causes neuronal supersentivity without receptor densensitization. J Pharmacol Exp Ther 1994; 268:595-599.
178. Herz A, Teschemacher HJ, Albus K et al. Morphine abstinence syndrome in rabbits precipitated by injection of morphine antagonists into the ventricular system and restricted parts of it. Psychopharmacologia 1972; 26:219-236.
179. Laschka E, Teschemacher P, Mehrain P et al. Sites of action of morphine involved in the development of physical dependence in rats. II. Morphine withdrawal precipitated by application of morphine antagonists into restricted parts of the ventricular system and by microinjection into various brain areas. Psychopharmacologia 1976; 46:141-147.
180. Wei E, Loh HH, Way EL. Neuroanatomical correlates of morphine dependence. Science 1972; 177:616-617.
181. Maldonado R, Fournié-Zaluski MC, Roques BP. Attenuation of the morphine withdrawal syndrome by inhibition of the endogenous enkephalin catabolism into the periaqueductal gray matter. Naunyn Schmiedebergs Arch Pharmacol 1992; 345:466-472.
182. Wei ET. Enkephalin analogs and physical dependence. J Pharmacol Exp Ther 1981; 216:12-18.
183. Sharpe LG, Garnett JE, Cicero TJ. Analgesia and hyperreactivity produced by intracranial microinjections of morphine into the periaqueductal gray matter of the rat. Behav Biol 1974; 11:303-313.
184. Jacquet YF, Lajtha A. The periaqueductal gray: Site of morphine analgesia and tolerance as shown by two-way cross-tolerance between systemic and intracerebral injections. Brain Res 1976; 103:501-513.
185. Vaccarino FJ, Bloom FE, Koob GF. Blockade of nucleus accumbens opiate receptors attenuates intravenous heroin reward in the rat. Psychopharmacology (Berlin) 1985; 85:37-42.
186. Higgings GA, Sellers EM. Antagonist-precipitated opioid withdrawal in rats: Evidence for dissociations between physical and motivational signs. Pharmacol Biochem Behav 1994; 48:1-8.
187. Harris GC, Aston-Jones G. Involvement of D_2 dopamine receptors in the nucleus accumbens in the opiate withdrawal syndrome. Nature 1994; 371:155-157.
188. Chahl LA, Thornton CA, Corliss A. Enhancement by haloperidol of the locomotor response induced by naloxone in morphine-treated guinea pigs. Neurosci Lett 1989; 96:213-217.

189. Brent PJ, Chahl LA. Enhancement of the opiate withdrawal response by antipsychotic drugs in guinea pigs is not mediated by sigma binding sites. Eur J Neuropsychopharmacol 1993; 3:23-32.

190. Kerr FWL, Pozuelo J. Suppression of physical dependence and induction of hypersensitivity to morphine by sterotaxic hypothalamic lesions in addicted rats. A new theory of addiction. Mayo Clin Proc 1971; 46:653-665.

191. Wikler A, Norrell H, Miller D. Limbic system and opioid addiction in the rat. Exp Neurol 1972; 34:543-557.

192. Le Gal la Salle G, Lagowska J. Amygdaloid kindling procedure reduces severity of morphine withdrawal syndrome in rats. Brain Res 1980; 184:239-242.

193. Tremblay EC, Charton G. Anatomical correlates of morphine withdrawal syndrome: Differential participation of structures located within the limbic system and striatum. Neurosci Lett 1981; 23:137-142.

194. Adler MW, Geller EB, Beeton PB et al. Inability of acute or chronic thalamic, limbic, or cortical lesions to alter narcotic dependence and abstinence in rats. Dev Neurosci 1978; 4:51-52.

195. Wei E, Tseng LF, Loh HH et al. Similarity of morphine abstinence signs to thermoregulatory behaviour. Nature 1974; 247: 398-340.

196. Kerr FWL. The role of the lateral hypothalamus in opiate dependence. In: Zimmermann E, George R, eds. Narcotics and the Hypothalmus. New York: Raven Press, 1974:23-35.

197. Lomax P, Ary M. Sites of action of narcotic analgesics in the hypothalamus. In: Zimmerman E, George R, eds. Narcotics and the Hypothalamus. New York: Raven Press, 1974:37-47.

198. Baumeister AA, Anticich TG, Hebert G et al. Evidence that physical dependence on morphine is mediated by the ventral midbrain. Neuropharmacology 1989; 28:1151-1157.

199. Baumeister AA, Richard AL, Richmond-Landeche L et al. Further studies of the role of opioid receptors in the nigra in the morphine withdrawal syndrome. Neuropharmacology 1992; 31:835-841.

200. Bläsig J, Papeschi R, Gramsch C et al. Central serotonergic mechanisms and development of morphine dependence. Drug Alcohol Depend 1976; 1:221-232.

201. Bederson JB, Fields HL, Barbaro NM. Hyperalgesia during naloxone-precipitated withdrawal from morphine is associated with increased on-cell activity in the rostral ventromedial medulla. Somatosens Mot Res 1990; 7:185-203.

202. Yap C, Taylor D. Involvement of 5-HT2 receptors in the wet dog shake behavior induced by 5-hydroxytryptophan in the rat. Neuropharmacology 1983; 22:801-804.

203. Araki H, Uchiyama-Tsutuli Y, Aihara H et al. Effects of chronic administration of haloperidol, methamphetamine or cocaine on "wet dog shakes" elicited by stimulation of the rat hippocampus. Arch Int Pharmacodyn Ther 1989; 297:217-224.

204. Mitchell CL, Grimes LM, Hong JS. Granule cells in the ventral dentate gyrus are essential for kainic acid-induced wet dog shakes but not those induced by precipitated abstinence in morphine-dependent rats. Brain Res 1990; 511:338-340.

205. Isaacson RL, Lanthorn TH. Hippocampal involvement in the pharmacological induction of withdrawal-like behaviors. Fed Proc 1981; 40:1500-1512.

206. Buccafusco JJ. Cardiovascular changes during morphine withdrawal in the rat: Effects of clonidine. Pharmacol Biochem Behav 1983; 18:209-215.

207. Miyamoto Y, Takemori AE. Sites of action of naloxone in precipitating withdrawal jumping in morphine-dependent mice: Investigations by the ED50 value and CNS content of naloxone. Drug Alcohol Depend 1993; 32:163-167.

208. Miyamoto Y, Takemori AE. Relative involvement of supraspinal and spinal mu opioid receptors in morphine dependence in mice. Life Sci 1993; 52:1039-1044.

CHAPTER 6

TOLERANCE AND SENSITIZATION TO OPIATES: RELATIONSHIP TO WITHDRAWAL

TOLERANCE: DEFINITION AND THEORETICAL BACKGROUND

Tolerance is usually defined as a decreased response to a drug with repeated administration or the requirement for larger doses of a drug to produce the same effect. Two types of tolerance exist: dispositional and pharmacodynamic. Dispositional tolerance is the decreased response to a drug with repeated administration due to a reduction in the amount of drug at its site of action. Pharmacodynamic tolerance refers to changes in response to a drug that result from adaptive changes excluding changes in the disposition of the drug. Although there is some evidence that metabolism to opiate drugs can be enhanced in tolerant animals, most opiate tolerance is thought to be pharmacodynamic.[1,2]

Two major hypotheses have been generated to explain tolerance: a habituation hypothesis and a homeostatic adaptive hypothesis.[3] The habituation hypothesis proposes that drug tolerance is the result of the response to the drug diminishing with repeated presentation.[4] Here, the extent to which a stimulus elicits a response depends on the extent to which it is unexpected or surprising. Based on the model of habituation developed by Wagner,[5] this habituation theory proposes that if the stimulus is primed in short-term memory and thus is expected, it will be responded to less. The decrease in response (habituation or tolerance) can be produced by recent presentations of the stimulus (opiate; this would be nonassociative tolerance) or by presentation of stimuli that predict or have been associated with the drug (associative tolerance). This theory predicts that infrequent administrations of high doses of opiate will lead to situation-specific (associative) tolerance, and frequent administrations of similar high doses will lead to situation-independent (nonassociative) tolerance. In fact, high, frequent doses should actually inhibit the development of situation-specific tolerance based on the hypothesis that frequent administration of high doses will continuously prime the short-term memory and as a result block the development of associations between the drug and environmental stimuli, an observation that has been confirmed.[6]

The homeostatic adaptive hypothesis proposes that the initial acute effect of the drug is opposed or counteracted by homeostatic changes in systems that mediate the primary drug effects. There are many versions of homeostatic models.[7-10] Here, the drug event is hypothesized to act as an unconditioned stimulus (UCS) that elicits an unconditioned response (UCR). Pairings of the drug event with distinctive environmental stimuli result in the environmental stimuli that acquire the ability to elicit conditional responses (CRs). However, drug CRs are often opposite in direction to the observed drug effect or what appears to be the unconditioned responses to the drug. In an opponent process formulation, stimuli paired with the end of the UCS or acute drug action can acquire conditioned opponent process responses, and compensatory CRs may be considered as evidence for a rapid conditioning of the B process.[8,9] In the case of opiate analgesia, the CR is hypothesized to be a compensatory CR or drug-opposite CR, e.g., a compensatory hyperalgesic response. In contrast, a CR like an observed drug effect would result in sensitization with an increase in the maximal effect observed. Determination of which type of conditioned response will develop—a conditioned drug-like CR or what is called a compensatory CR—depends on identification of where the response is initiated.[11] Drug-induced opposite effects have been difficult to demonstrate, and one reason may be the complex compound contextual stimuli that have been used as conditional stimuli.[12] For example, use of more discrete, controlled stimuli presentation has resulted in significant morphine-induced hyperthermia in rats.[13]

Some attempts have been made to incorporate both the habituation and homeostatic models in the search for the neurobiological mechanisms of tolerance, including a formulation described as decremental and oppositional.[14] Here, processes that change the number or function of drug-sensitive receptors with continued drug exposure would represent decremental models. In contrast, where continued drug treatment recruits processes that oppose the initial acute effects of the drug, this would be an example of an oppositional model.

A recent extension of the oppositional model focuses on neuroadaptation and argues that a distinction can be made between adaptations occurring within a drug-sensitive system and adaptations that occur between interacting systems.[15] For a within-system adaptation, repeated drug administration would elicit an opposing reaction within the same system that the drug elicits its primary pharmacological actions. Examples of this type of adaptation for opiate tolerance would be changes in opioid peptide systems such as receptor downregulation or changes in intracellular messenger systems (see chapter 3). For a between-system adaptation, initial changes in primary drug-sensitive neurons would be opposed by adaptations in other systems. One possible example might be an activation of a neuronal system that acts in opposition to the opiate drugs such as the antiopiate neuropeptide FF systems (see chapter 5). Ultimately, however, all of these hypotheses basically fit a homeostatic model, and such a homeostatic model basically inextricably links tolerance and dependence (see Table 6.1).

TOLERANCE TO OPIATES IN HUMANS

Tolerance to opiates in humans develops differentially.[1,2] There may be dramatic tolerance to some actions, whereas other actions of opiates may be unchanged. Tolerance develops to the analgesic, euphorigenic, sedative and other central nervous system depressant effects and to the lethal effects of opiates. Some addicts can build

Table 6.1. Tolerance and dependence-linking of cellular and behavioral levels of analysis

Within-systems Adaptation
Primary cellular response element to the drug would itself adapt to neutralize the drug's effects; persistence of the opposing effects after the drug disappears would produce the withdrawal response.

Between-systems Adaptation
A different cellular system and separable molecular apparatus would be triggered by the changes in the primary drug response neurons and would produce adaptation and tolerance.

up to enormous doses such as 2 grams of morphine intravenously over a period of 2-3 hours without significant changes in blood pressure or heart rate. The lethal dose of morphine in a nontolerant individual is approximately 30 mg parenterally and 120 mg orally.[16]

Certain effects of opiates are resistant to tolerance. Subjects very tolerant to the lethal or respiratory depressant effects of opiates still continue to show sedation, miosis and constipation.[17] Patients taking opiates chronically remain constipated despite some tolerance to the effects of opiates on gastrointestinal motility.[2] The phenomenon of resistance to tolerance has been studied extensively in methadone-maintained individuals.[18] Partial tolerance develops to the depression of sexual behavior in methadone-maintained individuals.[17] Constipation continues in a large number of methadone-maintained individuals for up to 8 months, insomnia is observed in 10-20% of patients and excessive sweating in 50% of patients.

Tolerance to opiates is characterized by a shortening of the duration of action but also a decrease in intensity. The rate of tolerance development is dependent on not only the dose of the drug but also the pattern of use. With doses in the therapeutic range and intermittent use, it is possible to obtain the desired analgesic effect for an indefinite period. When the opiate is taken in a continuous pattern, significant tolerance develops. Cross-tolerance develops to a high degree with opiates as long as the opiates are acting through the same receptor subtype.

TOLERANCE TO OPIATES IN ANIMALS

Tolerance to most of the effects of opiates develops rapidly in laboratory animals and is usually reflected in a shift of the dose-effect function to the right. The most common dependent variable for studies of tolerance to opiates in the laboratory is analgesia. Morphine treatment in mice over a period of 20 days produced parallel shifts in the analgesia dose-effect function to the right using two different measures of analgesia[19] (see Fig. 6.1). A similar shift to the right was observed with hypothermia and lethality. However, there was no tolerance to the motor-activating effects of morphine. In fact, there was some evidence of a sensitization in the motor-activating effects[19] (see Fig. 6.1).

Robust tolerance has been observed for the discriminative stimulus effects of opiates in animals, suggesting parallels with the subjective reports of tolerance in humans.[3,20,21] Tolerance to the rewarding effects of opiates with continuous administration, as measured by conditioned place preference, has also been observed.[22]

The rate of development of tolerance depends on the frequency and the amount of drug treatment. For example, with locomotor activation in mice, more frequent injection intervals (every 8 hours) resulted in dramatic tolerance instead of sensitization, as can be seen in Figure 6.2.[23] With continuous infusion, tolerance to the analgesic effects of morphine can develop within 6-8 hours of infusion.[24] In this experiment, reversal of tolerance required more than 2 weeks.

Finally, it is important to note that both environment-dependent (associative) and environment-independent (nonassociative) tolerance have been demonstrated; this distinction is predicted by habituation theory.[4] As noted above, infrequent administration of high doses of opiates favors environment-dependent tolerance, whereas frequent administration of the same doses favors environment-independent tolerance.[6,25]

NEUROBIOLOGICAL SUBSTRATES FOR TOLERANCE

At the neurobiological level, the two hypotheses to explain tolerance parallel the theoretical positions described above. Habituation or decremental models of tolerance would presumably be reflected

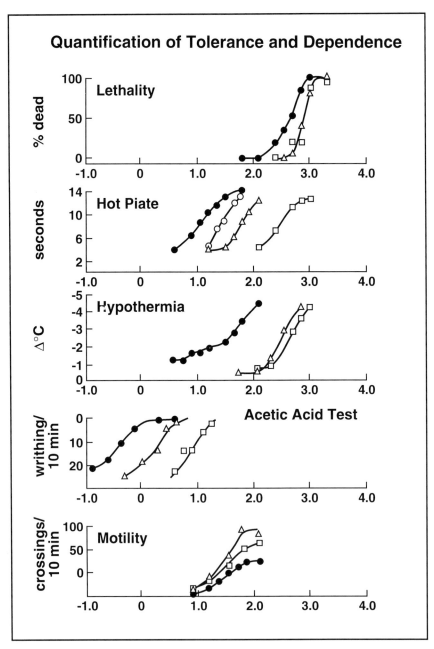

Fig. 6.1. Effects of morphine pretreatment on the dose-response functions for morphine
in five different measures in mice. Values represent dose-response curves to morphine-
HCL in different test situations. Solid circles: acute morphine; open circles: 1 x 16 mg/kg
for 20 days; open triangles: 1 x 64 mg/kg for 20 days; open squares: 2 x 128 mg/kg for
20 days. Each point represents the mean results from at least 15 animals. Horizontal axis
represents log mg/kg morphine-HCL. Reproduced with permission from Fernandes M et
al, Naunyn Schmiedebergs Arch Pharmacol 1977; 297:53-60.

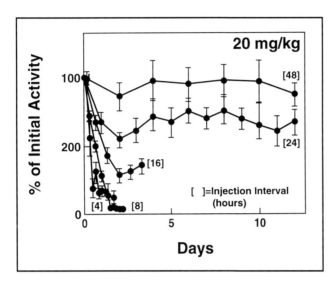

Fig. 6.2. Effects of multiple doses of an opiate on tolerance in mice. Levorphanol (20 mg/kg) was injected intraperitoneally at various intervals. Running activity was measured after each injection and is expressed as percent of initial activity for each group of mice. Numbers in the brackets represent the injection interval for each curve of 4, 8, 16, 24 and 48 hours. Reproduced with permission from Goldstein A et al, J Pharmacol Exp Ther 1969; 169:175-184.

in changes in the receptors to the drugs themselves. The homeostatic adaptive or oppositional model would predict that the effects of the opiate are antagonized by changes elsewhere in other biochemical pathways or other neuronal systems.

There is some evidence of receptor downregulation with opiates. In cultured neuroblastoma x glioma hybrid NG108-15 cells that express only δ-opiate receptors, exposure of these cells to opiates for several hours reduces the ability of these cells to inhibit adenylate cyclase,[26] and similar results have now been observed for the μ-receptor using prolactin-secreting rat pituitary tumor 7315c cells that express only μ-receptors.[27] In intact animals, no decrease in opiate receptor binding was observed using radioligands that bind to multiple opiate receptors.[28] However, using more selective radioligands, an approximately 30-40% decrease in selective μ-receptor binding was observed in the cortex of tolerant rats.[29] Some of these receptor downregulation effects have been linked to a decrease or loss of a physiological response.[30] Another mechanism by which receptor function could become decreased with chronic drug exposure is by a functional decoupling from G-proteins involved in signal transduction. Some evidence exists to show that in the locus coeruleus, opiates lose their ability to increase potassium conductance, which presumably depends on G-protein activation, and thus lose their ability to decrease firing with chronic administration.[31] Finally, at the system level, a feedback inhibition hypothesis would predict that chronic opiate treatment would produce feedback inhibition of endogenous opioid systems. Some evidence for decreased biosynthesis of pro-opiomelanocortin has been observed with chronic opiate treatment,[32] but increases in striatal prodynorphin have also been observed with chronic opiate treatment.[33] Thus, some evidence exists for molecular, cellular and system support of the habituation model, but this is not the only neurobiological mechanism implicated in tolerance.

Oppositional or homeostatic adaptive mechanisms have been identified at the molecular, cellular and system level to explain tolerance,[15] and these changes can be within-system or between-system. A good example of a molecular within-system change is the changes in adenylate cyclase that occur in vitro in NG108-15 cells. Acute administration of morphine inhibits adenylate cyclase, and with chronic treatment this inhibition declines. Removal of the opiate or precipitated withdrawal results in adenylate cyclase above normal levels (see chapter 3). These changes occur over days and thus have a different time course than desensitization which occurs more rapidly.

Thus, inhibition by an opiate of second messenger system function could lead to tolerance and dependence through a compensating "hypertrophy" in this same system,[34] as described in chapter 3. The neuroblastoma x glioma hybrid cell (NG108-15 cells), cultured in the presence of an opiate, develops tolerance and dependence as reflected in an increased production of cyclic AMP under certain situations.[35,36] Again, as described in detail in chapter 3, there is significant other support for the hypothesis of an activation of cyclic AMP in the neurons of dependent animals, and subsequent studies have extended the early whole brain and in vitro biochemical studies to specific structures in the central nervous system that have been implicated in opiate withdrawal such as the locus coeruleus (see chapter 3). Acute morphine decreases the activity of the second messenger system (e.g., cyclic AMP system in the locus coeruleus) at all levels of biochemical transduction of the physiological response, and chronic morphine upregulates the cyclic AMP system at every major step between receptor and response,[37-39] including protein kinase[38] and G-proteins[37] (see Fig. 3.1, chapter 3).

The next step in these intracellular pathways, the regulation by second messengers of protein phosphorylation, provides a further means of explaining the neuroadaptation associated with opiate tolerance. Again, as described in chapter 3, many types of proteins are regulated by phosphorylation including phosphorylation of cytoskeletal proteins which affects the size and shape of neurons and phosphorylation of nuclear proteins which affects their ability to regulate gene expression. These changes presumably include those that may trigger the longer-term effects of the drugs that eventually lead to tolerance.

At the cellular level, there are some studies demonstrating "between-system" compensating responses where other neurotransmitter systems are recruited that may blunt the acute effects of opiates and result in tolerance. A series of elegant studies of cellular mechanisms of nociception have provided a model of the type of between-systems adaptation that could also contribute to tolerance.[40,41] There are nociceptive modulatory neurons in the rostral ventromedial medulla—"on-cells"—that are depressed by morphine administration but show firing bursts just prior to the actual tail-flick reflex. This on-cell activity correlates well with hyperalgesia. In contrast, "off-cells" in the rostral ventromedial medulla are excited by morphine but are silent or inactive during naloxone-precipitated hyperalgesia.[40] Opioid peptides and opiates appear to increase the firing of off-cells by inhibiting the on-cell GABA inhibition,[41] suggesting that the hyperalgesic opponent response may involve an enhanced GABAergic transmission.

This neuroadaptation is by no means the only cellular example for a model of a between-systems oppositional mechanism. Recent evidence suggests both within-system and between-system adaptations in the functional activity of the locus coeruleus and its inputs during opiate withdrawal.[42,43] Also, at the molecular level, chronic opiate administration is also associated with changes in second messenger systems in the mesocorticolimbic dopamine system[39] (see chapter 3).

At the system level, it is clear that a number of neurotransmitter systems may act in opposition to opiate peptides to produce a between-system tolerance. Recent evidence suggests that neuropeptide FF, CCK or dynorphin may be activated with chronic opiates (see chapter 5). For example, morphine, even acutely, can stimulate neuropeptide FF release in rat spinal cord slices, and in vivo a single administration of heroin can cause a decrease in spinal neuropeptide FF content.[44] In addition, glutamate systems have been implicated in opiate tolerance, since the development of tolerance to the analgesic effects of morphine can be prevented by administration of N-methyl-D-aspartate (NMDA) receptor antagonists.[33] Clearly, at this level of analysis there would be strong evidence implicating the same between-system adaptations associated with withdrawal with the development of tolerance[15] (see chapters 5 and 8).

SENSITIZATION

Sensitization has been defined as: "the long-lasting increment in response occurring upon repeated presentation of a stimulus that reliably elicits a response at its initial presentation"[45] or "the increased response to a drug that follows its repeated intermittent presentation."[46] As with tolerance, sensitization of a drug effect can be linked to stimuli or events that occurred when the original effect was elicited, often termed environment-dependent sensitization.[47] Sensitization is more likely to occur with intermittent exposure to a drug, in contrast to tolerance which is more likely to occur with continuous exposure.

Repeated intermittent administration of opiate drugs can lead to long-lasting sensitization to the behavioral activating effects of opiates,[48] and some of these effects can last up to 240 days after ceasing the treatment.[49] In an early study, the rats were treated with 20 mg/kg of morphine injected intraperitoneally (IP) for 59 days and locomotor activity tested for 7 hours after treatment using jiggle cage actometers. The initial depression in activity underwent tolerance within 4-6 days and then gradually changed into excitation (Figs. 6.3 and 6.4). This initial depression returned after cessation of chronic treatment; however, the excitation remained sensitized (Fig. 6.4). This dichotomy was confirmed in dose-response challenge studies where it was shown that a low dose of morphine (1.25 mg/kg) administered repeatedly in rats that had been made dependent on morphine 80 mg/kg/day showed only the excitatory effect and sensitization persisted unchanged 160 days

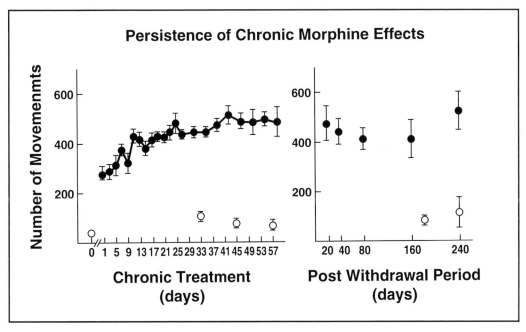

Fig. 6.3. Effects of 20 mg/kg injected IP of morphine HCL upon locomotor activity of rats at the third hour of recording following chronic daily treatment for 59 days. Reproduced with permission from Babbini M et al, Neuropharmacology 1975; 14:611-614.

later.[50] In dose-effect studies of the chronically administered drug, the amount of drug-induced hyperactivity appeared to be directly related to the dose of the preceding chronic treatment[51] (Fig. 6.5). Cross-sensitization was observed to methadone but not meperidine,[52] suggesting that some aspect of the meperidine discriminative stimulus is different and can influence the sensitization process. This may have been an early indication of what is now termed environment-dependent sensitization where, in this case, the environment is an internal cue.

While an early study failed to show a cross-sensitization of opiates to amphetamine,[53] subsequent studies have shown an increase in locomotor activity to systemic amphetamine after a history of systemic morphine.[54] Differences in the two studies may be related to the dose of morphine during the pretreatment phase. In the Babbini study, the animals were treated daily for 26 days with 20 mg/kg of morphine;[53] in the Stewart and Vezina study, the animals received 10 mg/kg morphine on four occasions. In this study, a higher dose of 20 mg/kg did not lead to cross-sensitization.[54] Perhaps more important for understanding the neural basis

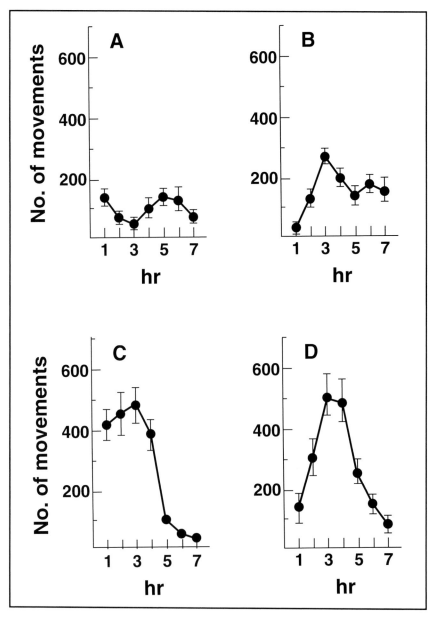

Fig. 6.4. Time-effect functions of 20 mg/kg of morphine injected IP on locomotor activity of rats. A: saline; B: morphine, first day; C: morphine after 58 days of daily treatment; D: morphine 8 months after the termination of chronic treatment. Reproduced with permission from Babbini M et al, Neuropharmacology 1975; 14: 611-614.

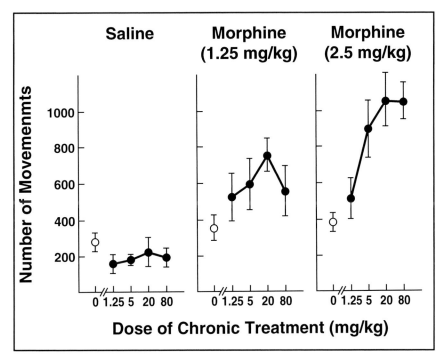

Fig. 6.5. Effects of morphine (1.25 and 2.5 mg/kg IP) on locomotor activity in nondependent rats (open circles) or in animals previously treated chronically with various doses of morphine (solid black circles). Reproduced with permission from Bartoletti M et al, Neuropharmacology 1987; 26:115-119.

of opiate sensitization, these authors also observed a cross-sensitization of systemic morphine to the direct injection of opioids into the ventral tegmental area dopamine system. These results suggested a role for the mesolimbic dopamine system not only in the sensitization associated with psychomotor stimulants such as amphetamine but also in the sensitization associated with opiate drugs.

Again, sensitization also has environment-dependent and environment-independent components. Animals exposed repeatedly to a drug in the presence of a given set of environmental cues will, when given the test for sensitization, show a greater response to the drug than animals exposed to the drug in a different environment.[46] In fact, with morphine injections into the ventral tegmental area, sensitization only occurred in the environment that had been paired with the morphine injections.[55] However, in subsequent experiments where amphetamine was injected into the ventral

tegmental area, presumably at a dose sufficient to cause somatodendritic release of dopamine, cross-sensitization to systemic morphine occurred regardless of the environmental pairings, suggesting the existence of environment-independent (nonassociative)
sensitization.[56]

Several explanations have been proposed for the apparent environmental control over sensitization. An operant conditioning
hypothesis is that the control over the expression of sensitization
may be due to differences in the training environments,[57] and different behavioral patterns are operantly conditioned in each environment. An alternative hypothesis is a Pavlovian model where
the salience of the conditioned stimulus may play an important
role. As in the latent inhibition phenomena associated with learning, familiarization with specific environmental cues retards the
development of their association with a given drug effect. Here,
the stressful properties of the novel test environment contribute to
environment-dependent sensitization and may depend on activation of some part of the stress axis. For example, with psychomotor stimulants, sensitization is greater if amphetamine is given
in a novel environment as opposed to a familiar home cage
environment.[58]

Sensitization has also been observed to the rewarding effects of
opiates. In an early observation, rats trained on a fixed-interval
schedule (fixed interval 2 minutes) and subjected to twice daily
injections of morphine of 40 mg/kg IP showed a rapid tolerance
to the rate-decreasing effects of morphine and a progressive increase in lever-pressing compared to control rats that persisted for
the duration of the morphine treatment period. One interpretation of these results is that the reinforcing effects of morphine
have become sensitized with repeated administration. Similarly,
studies with drug discrimination have shown that pre-exposure to
opiates can shift the drug discrimination dose-effect function to
the left.[59,60] However, chronic continuous opiate exposure has the
opposite effect in trained animals, shifting the dose-effect function
to the right.[20]

Repeated prior exposure to morphine also increased the drug's
rewarding effects as measured in the conditioned place preference
test.[61] However, tolerance to the rewarding effects of opiates was

also observed using conditioned place preference when the animals were exposed to the drug continuously prior to place conditioning training.[22] Again, the differences in history of drug exposure, frequency of administration and dose are critical in determining whether one observes sensitization or tolerance. Chronic continuous administration clearly favors tolerance (see above); intermittent exposure with an appropriately long period between the test dose and previous dosing favors sensitization.

ACUTE DEPENDENCE: SENSITIZATION TO PRECIPITATED WITHDRAWAL

Studies with human subjects have suggested that adaptive changes in response to administration of opiates may begin with a single exposure. For example, administration of an opiate antagonist such as naloxone following pretreatment with a single dose of morphine or methadone results in physiological signs, subjective ratings and objective (somatic) symptoms characteristic of withdrawal from chronic opiates.[62-70] This phenomenon has been referred to as "acute dependence,"[63,71] which can be defined operationally as "a state in which abstinence can be demonstrated or precipitated following either a single dose or a short-term infusion of morphine." Others in describing this phenomenon in animals have variably used the terms "single-dose dependence" (e.g., Meyer and Sparber[72]), "acute sensitization" of antagonist effects (e.g., White-Gbadebo and Holtzman[73,74]), and "acute withdrawal" (e.g., Cohen et al[75]), although "acute dependence" is by far the most commonly used term.

The severity of naloxone-precipitated withdrawal in the human model of acute dependence varies as a function of the dose of opiate agonist,[63,67] the dose of antagonist[64] and the interval between agonist pretreatment and naloxone administration, with abstinence signs being observed when naloxone is given as soon as 45 minutes or as late as 24 hours after a single dose of morphine.[65,66,69] Furthermore, the intensity of naloxone-precipitated withdrawal signs increases progressively with repeated exposure to morphine.[62,68] This increase in naloxone-precipitated withdrawal severity has been observed in subjects with no prior history of opiate use or abuse,[62] providing evidence that adaptive changes in response to opiate treatment can be seen following the very first exposure to the opiate and can increase progressively with repeated intermittent exposure.

The observation of acute dependence as defined by antagonist precipitation of *somatic* withdrawal signs following acute pretreatment with opiates has been reported in a number of species other than humans, including monkeys, dogs, gerbils, mice and rats.[71,76-84] In many of these studies, *high doses* of agonist and/or antagonist were typically employed to demonstrate a significant incidence of somatic withdrawal signs. In dogs, however, naloxone (3 mg/kg) elicited clear signs of opiate withdrawal when the animals were pretreated intravenously with *0.1 mg/kg of morphine* 1.5 hours earlier, suggesting that this phenomenon can be observed following relatively small doses of opiate agonists.[79] Recently, a variety of somatic signs of withdrawal were elicited by low-moderate doses of naloxone (0.1-0.3 mg/kg) administered 4 hours following a single morphine exposure (5 mg/kg), and these signs were more prevalent following a second morphine exposure.[85]

Acute dependence in humans not only involves somatic physical signs but also a number of subjective affective signs. In animal models of the negative affective consequences of opiate withdrawal, increased potency of opiate antagonists to suppress operant response rates and elevate brain stimulation reward thresholds can also be observed following treatment with a *single dose* of morphine in rats. This phenomenon may reflect the initial adaptive changes leading to the development of a state of chronic opiate dependence.[72,85-87] Furthermore, repeated intermittent exposure to moderate doses of morphine results in progressive increases in the magnitude of antagonist effects, suggesting a form of sensitization.[85-89] More recently, there is evidence that naltrexone dose-dependently elevates brain stimulation reward thresholds in rats treated acutely with morphine,[88] similar to what is seen in withdrawal from chronic opiate treatment.[90,91] Thus, opiate antagonists administered after acute administration of morphine can produce effects (somatic withdrawal-like signs, suppression of operant responding for food, altered brain reward thresholds) which are reminiscent of the antagonist-precipitated withdrawal syndrome seen in chronically dependent rats. These effects get larger with subsequent challenges and can last up to 6 weeks,[85] showing parallels to other forms of sensitization phenomena.

NEUROBIOLOGICAL SUBSTRATES FOR SENSITIZATION

Sensitization to the locomotor activating effects of opiates appears to involve and may depend on activation of the mesolimbic dopamine system. Injections of opiates directly into the ventral tegmental area show sensitized responses in animals previously made dependent,[92] and injection of opioid peptides directly into the ventral tegmental area also produces sensitization.[93] At low doses of opioid peptides there is no evidence of an initial hypoactivity.[93] Repeated microinjections of amphetamine into the somatodendritic region of the ventral tegmental area dopamine cells, at doses that do not cause behavioral activation, are sufficient to produce sensitization to later systemic injections of amphetamine or morphine. Thus, it is likely that changes in the functioning of these cells are sufficient to produce sensitization.[56,94]

The exact mechanism of action for sensitization to opiates is largely unknown, but there are substantial clues for the mechanism of action for the locomotor activating effects that can be found in the psychomotor stimulant literature. While multiple mechanisms have been proposed, a common theme is that there is a time-dependent chain of adaptations that lead ultimately to the long-lasting changes associated with locomotor sensitization.[95,96] Repeated administration of cocaine produces a decrease in the sensitivity of impulse-regulating somatodendritic dopamine D-2 autoreceptors, which would translate into enhanced dopaminergic function with subsequent injections.[97] There are some difficulties with this explanation as the sole dopaminergic mechanism for sensitization. For example, there are differences in the time course of dopaminergic subsensitivity; it disappears within 4-8 days, and sensitization can persist for weeks.[98] Sensitization can also be blocked by D-1 antagonists,[99] although sensitization persists in D-1 knockout mice.[100] Also, while amphetamine injected into the nucleus accumbens fails to produce sensitization,[101] direct dopamine agonists can produce sensitization in dopamine-denervated animals.[102]

In addition, there appears to be an important role for a stress connection in sensitization.[103] Activation of the corticotropin releasing factor (CRF) brain system and activation of the hypothalamic pituitary adrenal axis have been shown to be permissive for psychomotor stimulant sensitization. Stressors can cause sensitization to stimulant drugs, and there appears to be an important role for extrahypothalamic CRF in stress-induced sensitization.[104]

Finally, glutamate systems have also been implicated in behavioral sensitization to amphetamine and cocaine. Blockade of N-methyl-D-aspartate receptors blocks the development of sensitization to these psychomotor stimulants.[105-108] This glutamate antagonism appears to block both environment-dependent and environment-independent sensitization.[109]

Thus the mesolimbic dopamine system and its modulation by glutamate receptors, CRF and the hypothalamic pituitary adrenal axis play an important role in psychomotor stimulant sensitization. The specific role of mesolimbic autoreceptors and stress in opiate sensitization could provide a focus for future hypothesis testing.

TOLERANCE, SENSITIZATION AND WITHDRAWAL

Tolerance and sensitization (reverse tolerance) can be observed with many of the effects of opiate drugs, and at first glance it is difficult to understand how both processes can result from repeated drug exposure and how they both contribute to withdrawal and dependence. There are clearly a number of factors that contribute to the manifestation of one or the other phenomena. The nature of the dependent variable is critical. Tolerance readily develops to the analgesic and response-suppressing (sedative) effects of opiates, and one is hard pressed to observe sensitization to these two measures (see above). In contrast, the activating effects of opiates readily show sensitization, although tolerance has been observed particularly with high doses and continuous administration (see above). A similar pattern to the locomotor-activating effects has been observed for the rewarding effects in animals. Interestingly, sensitization can also occur to the acute dependence effects of opiates as measured by naloxone-precipitated withdrawal. The route of administration, dosing procedure and dose all play a role in determining whether tolerance or sensitization will occur with continuous administration of high doses favoring tolerance and intermittent dosing favoring sensitization. However, it is important to note that even dependent animals show sensitization to the behavioral activating effects of opiates if enough days are allowed to elapse post-dependence, and that this sensitized locomotor response remains even up to 8 months post-dependence (Fig. 6.4).

The question remains as to what the relationship is between tolerance, sensitization and withdrawal. One can invoke an adaptive homeostatic hypothesis to explain the coexistence of both phenomena as part of an attempt of the body to return to an equilibrium state. Tolerance to the analgesic effects of opiates could be considered to reflect an underlying hyperalgesia to counteract the externally induced analgesia. This rebound phenomenon would be one component of opiate withdrawal. The difficulty with this position has been the difficulty in measuring the rebound hyperalgesia,[12] although recent studies have observed such phenomena both at the behavioral[44,110] and cellular[41] levels. Also, the actual mechanism by which the withdrawal effects, e.g., acute dependence, become sensitized remains to be determined.

Locomotor activation that becomes sensitized is more problematic for an adaptive homeostatic position. The sedative actions of opiates clearly mask the activating effects when large doses of opiates are used, and low, nonsedative doses do not show sensitization.[48] However, opiates, even after the first injection, can produce robust locomotor activation when directly injected into the ventral tegmental area, and sensitization can still occur to these nonsedative-influenced injections,[93] thus requiring some unknown source of inhibition to satisfy an adaptive hypothesis.

Another alternative is that sensitization is, in fact, a secondary response to the original adaptive response. Thus, there would be an activation of the mesolimbic dopamine system induced by endogenous neurochemical mechanisms that were caused by the initial attempt of the body to adapt to the drug insult. In terms of the opponent process theory (see chapter 8) this would be, in effect, a second A process that follows the B process in a sort of ripple effect. Thus, to use a simplistic schema, acute morphine would acutely stimulate a release of dopamine followed by the engagement of mechanisms to decrease the increased dopaminergic activity (again, a relatively short-term response) followed by the sensitized response which would be a long-term reaction to that decrease. This might also explain the sensitization seen in acute dependence. A secondary exaggerated morphine response after the second injection (secondary A process) would produce an even greater aversive effect (secondary B process) upon a second morphine naloxone challenge. Unexplained at this time is why or how the sensitized response remains for such a long period. In the case of dependent animals it appears to be virtually permanent.

To summarize, chronic administration of opiates produces tolerance and sensitization to subsequent morphine challenges. Tolerance is more likely to occur to the analgesic and sedative effects of opiates and sensitization is more likely to occur to the activating and rewarding effects of opiates, although tolerance is also seen in these effects with high doses and continuous administration. Intermittent administration favors the development of sensitization in the absence of tolerance, and continuous administration favors the development of tolerance in the absence of overt sensitization. Two major hypotheses have been developed to explain tolerance to drugs and opiates in particular: habituation and homeostatic counteradaptation. Habituation theory can explain the lack of obvious compensatory responses but falls short in terms of neurobiological mechanisms. Homeostatic counteradaptation theory has many strengths including some solid neurobiological evidence and a clear link to withdrawal. However, homeostatic counteradaptation falls short in that many times the hypothesized counteradaptation has not been identified. Sensitization has a neurobiological explanation for changes in the modulation of the mesolimbic dopamine system but requires some conceptual somersaults to integrate with counteradaptation theory. Future studies at the molecular, cellular and systems levels will undoubtedly provide significant insight into these issues.

REFERENCES

1. Jaffe JH. Drug addiction and drug use. In: Gilman AG, Rall TW, Nies AS et al, eds. Goodman and Gilman's The Pharmacological Basis of Therapeutics. 8th ed. New York: Pergamon Press, 1990:522-573.

2. Jaffe JH, Martin WR. Opioid analgesics and antagonists. In: Gilman AG, Rall TW, Nies AS et al, eds. Goodman and Gilman's The Pharmacological Basis of Therapeutics. 8th ed. New York: Pergamon Press, 1990:485-521.

3. Young AM, Goudie AJ. Adaptive processes regulating tolerance to the behavioral effects of drugs. In: Bloom FE, Kupfer DJ, eds. Psychopharmacology: The Fourth Generation of Progress. New York: Raven Press, Ltd., 1995:733-742.

4. Baker TB, Tiffany ST. Morphine tolerance as habituation. Psychol Rev 1985; 92:78-108.

5. Wagner AR. Priming in STM: An information processing mechanism for self-generated or retrieval-generated depression in performance. In: Tighe TJ, Leaton RN, eds. Habituation: Perspectives from child development, animal behavior and neurophysiology. Hillsdale, NJ: Lawrence Erlbaum, 1976:95-128.

6. Tiffany ST, Drobes DJ, Cepeda-Benito A. Contribution of associative and nonassociative processes to the development of morphine tolerance. Psychopharmacology 1992; 109:185-190.

7. Solomon RL, Corbit JD. An opponent-process theory of motivation: 1. Temporal dynamics of affect. Psychol Rev 1974; 81: 119-145.

8. Siegel S. Evidence from rats that morphine tolerance is a learned response. J Comp Physiol Psychol 1975; 89:498-506.

9. Solomon RL. The opponent-process theory of acquired motivation: The affective dynamics of addiction. In: Maser JD, Seligman MEP, eds. Psychopathology: Experimental Models. San Francisco: W.H. Freeman and Co., 1977:124-145.

10. Poulos CX, Cappell H. Homeostatic theory of drug tolerance: A general model of physiological adaptation. Psychol Rev 1991; 98:390-408.

11. Stewart J, De Wit H, Eikelboom R. Role of unconditioned and conditioned drug effects in the self-admininstration of opiates and stimulants. Psychol Rev 1984; 91:251-268.

12. Goudie AJ. Conditioned opponent processes in the development of tolerance to psychoactive drugs. Prog Neuropsych Biol Psych 1990; 14:675-688.

13. Cunningham CL, Schwartz KS. Pavlovian-conditioned changes in body temperature induced by alcohol and morphine. Drug Dev Res 1989; 16:295-303.

14. Littleton JM, Little HJ. Adaptation in neuronal calcium channels as a common basis for physical dependence on central depressant drugs. In: Goudie AJ, Emmett-Oglesby MW, eds. Psychoactive Drugs: Tolerance and Sensitization. Clifton, NJ: Humana Press, 1989:461-518.

15. Koob GF, Bloom FE. Cellular and molecular mechanisms of drug dependence. Science 1988; 242:715-723.
16. Ellenhorn MJ, Barceloux DG. Medical Toxicology. New York: Elsevier, 1988.
17. Martin WR, Jasinski DR, Haertzen CA et al. Methadone—A re-evaluation. Arch Gen Psychiatry 1973; 28:286-295.
18. Kreek MJ. Pharmacologic modalities of therapy: Methadone maintenance and the use of narcotic antagonists. In: Stimmel B, ed. Heroin Dependency. New York: Stratton Intercontinental Medical Book Corp., 1975:232-294.
19. Fernandes M, Kluwe S, Coper H. Quantitative assessment of tolerance to and dependence on morphine in mice. Naunyn Schmiedebergs Arch Pharmacol 1977; 297:53-60.
20. Young AM, Sannerud CA, Steigerwald ES et al. Tolerance to morphine stimulus control: Role of morphine maintenance dose. Psychopharmacology 1990; 102:59-67.
21. Young AM, Walton MA, Carter TL. Selective tolerance to discriminative stimulus effects of morphine or d-amphetamine. Behav Pharmacol 1992; 3:201-209.
22. Shippenberg TS, Emmett-Oglesby MW, Ayesta FJ et al. Tolerance and selective cross-tolerance to the motivational effects of opioids. Psychopharmacology 1988; 96:110-115.
23. Goldstein A, Sheehan P. Tolerance to opioid narcotics. I. Tolerance to the "running fit" caused by levorphanol in the mouse. J Pharmacol Exp Ther 1969; 169:175-184.
24. Cox BM, Ginsburg M, Osman OH. Acute tolerance to the narcotic analgesic drugs in rats. Br J Pharmacol 1968; 33:245-256.
25. Dafters R, Odber J. Effects of dose, interdose interval and drug-signal parameters on morphine analgesic tolerance: Implications for current theories of tolerance. Behav Neurosci 1989; 103:1082-1090.
26. Sharma SK, Klee WA, Nirenberg M. Opiate-dependent modulation of adenylate cyclase. Proc Natl Acad Sci USA 1977; 74:3365-3369.
27. Puttfarcken PS, Werling LL, Cox BM. Effects of chronic morphine exposure on opioid inhibition of adenylyl cyclase in 7315c cell membranes: A useful model for the study of tolerance at mu opioid receptors. Mol Pharmacol 1988; 33:520-527.
28. Cox BM. Drug tolerance and physical dependence. In: Pratt WB, Taylor P, eds. Principles of Drug Action, The Basis of Pharmacology. 3rd ed. New York: Churchill Livingstone, 1990:639-689.
29. Werling LL, McMahon PN, Cox BM. Selective changes in mu receptor properties induced by chronic morphine exposure. Proc Natl Acad Sci USA 1989; 86:6394-6397.
30. Dingledine R, Valentino RJ, Bostock E et al. Downregulation of

delta but not mu opioid receptors in the hippocampal slice associated with loss of physiological response. Life Sci 1983; 33(Suppl 1):333-336.

31. Christies MJ, Williams JT, North RA. Cellular mechanisms of opioid tolerance: Studies in single brain neurons. Mol Pharmacol 1987; 32:633-638.

32. Bronstein DM, Przewlocki R, Akil H. Effects of morphine treatment on pro-opio-melanocortin systems in rat brain. Brain Res 1990; 519:102-111.

33. Trujillo KA, Akil H. Opiate tolerance and dependence: Recent finding and synthesis. The New Biologist 1991; 3:915-923.

34. Collier HOJ. Cellular site of opiate dependence. Nature 1980; 283:625-630.

35. Sharma SK, Klee WA, Nirenberg M. Dual regulation of adenylate cyclase accounts for narcotic dependence and tolerance. Proc Natl Acad Sci USA 1975; 72:3092-3096.

36. Traber J, Gullis R, Hamprecht B. Influence of opiates on the levels of adenosine 3'5'-cyclic monophosphate in neuroblastoma x glioma hybrid cells. Life Sci 1975; 16:1863-1868.

37. Nestler EJ, Erdos JJ, Terwilliger R et al. Regulation of G-proteins by chronic morphine in the rat locus coeruleus. Brain Res 1989; 476:230-239.

38. Nestler EJ, Tallman JF. Chronic morphine treatment increases cyclic AMP-dependent protein kinase activity in the rat locus coeruleus. Mol Pharmacol 1988; 33:127-132.

39. Nestler EJ. Molecular mechanisms of drug addiction. J Neurosci 1992; 12:2439-2450.

40. Kim DH, Fields HL, Barbaro NM. Morphine analgesia and acute physical dependence: Rapid onset of two opposing dose-related processes. Brain Res 1990; 516:37-40.

41. Fields HL, Heinricher MM, Mason P. Neurotransmitters in nociceptive modulatory circuits. Annu Rev Neurosci 1991; 14:219-245.

42. Akaoka H, Aston-Jones G. Opiate withdrawal-induced hyperactivity of locus coeruleus neurons is substantially mediated by augmented excitatory acid input. J Neurosci 1991; 11:3830-3839.

43. Koob GF, Markou A, Weiss F et al. Opponent process and drug dependence: Neurobiological mechanisms. Semin Neurosci 1993; 5:351-358.

44. Devillers J-P, Boisserie F, Laulin J-P et al. Simultaneous activation of spinal antiopioid system (neuropeptide FF) and pain facilitatory circuitry by stimulation of opioid receptors in rats. Brain Res 1995; 700:173-181.

45. Groves PM, Thompson RF. Habituation: A dual-process theory. Psychol Rev 1970; 77:419-450.

46. Stewart J, Badiani A. Tolerance and sensitization to the behavioral effects of drugs. Behav Pharmacol 1993; 4:289-312.

47. Stewart J. Conditioned stimulus control of the expression of sensitization of the behavioral activating effects of opiate and stimulant drugs. In: Gormezano I, Wasserman EA, eds. Learning and Memory: Behavioral and Biological Substrates. Hillsdale, NJ: Lawrence Erlbaum, 1992:129-151.

48. Babbini M, Davis WM. Time-dose relationship for locomotor activity effects of morphine after acute or repeated treatment. Br J Pharmacol 1972; 46:213-224.

49. Babbini M, Gaiardi M, Bartoletti M. Persistence of chronic morphine effects upon activity in rats 8 months after ceasing the treatment. Neuropharmacology 1975; 14:611-614.

50. Bartoletti M, Giardi M, Gubellini C et al. Long-term sensitization to the excitatory effects of morphine. Neuropharmacology 1983; 22:1193-1196.

51. Bartoletti M, Gairdi M, Gubellini C et al. Previous treatment with morphine and sensitization to the excitatory actions of opiates: Dose-effect relationships. Neuropharmacology 1987; 26:115-119.

52. Bartoletti M, Giardi M, Gubellini C et al. Cross-sensitization to the excitatory effect of morphine in post-dependent rats. Neuropharmacology 1985; 24:889-893.

53. Babbini M, Gaiardi M, Bartoletti M. Motility effects of methamphetamine in rats chronically treated with morphine. Neuropharmacology 1978; 17:979-983.

54. Vezina P, Giovino AA, Wise RA et al. Environment-specific cross-sensitization between the locomotor activating effects of morphine and amphetamine. Pharmacol Biochem Behav 1989; 32:581-584.

55. Vezina P, Stewart J. Conditioning and place-specific sensitization of increases in activity induced by morphine in the VTA. Pharmacol Biochem Behav 1984; 20:925-934.

56. Vezina P, Stewart J. Amphetamine administered to the ventral tegmental area but not the nucleus accumbens sensitizes rats to systemic morphine: Lack of conditioned effects. Brain Res 1990; 516:99-106.

57. Willner P, Papp M, Cheeta S et al. Environmental influences on behavioural sensitization to the dopamine agonist quinpirole. Behav Pharmacol 1992; 3:43-50.

58. Badiani A, Robinson TE. Enhancement of amphetamine sensitization in a novel environment: The role of adrenal hormones. In: Seredenin SB, Longo V, Gaviraghi G, eds. Biological Basis of Individual Sensitivity to Psychotropic Drugs. Edinburgh, UK: Graffhan Press Ltd., 1994:231-241.

59. Gaiardi M, Bartoletti M, Gubellini C et al. Sensitivity to the nar-

cotic cue in non-dependent and post-dependent rats. Neuro-pharmacology 1986; 25:119-123.

60. Gubellini C, Bacchi A, Gaiardi M et al. Sensitivity to the narcotic cue in rats repeatedly exposed to morphine before discrimination training. Pharmacol Res 1990; 22(Suppl 1):115-116.

61. Lett BT. Repeated exposures intensify rather than diminish the re-warding effects of amphetamine, morphine and cocaine. Psychop-harmacology 1989; 98:357-362.

62. Azorlosa JL, Stitzer ML, Greenwald MK. Opioid physical depen-dence development: Effects of single versus repeated morphine pre-treatments and of subjects' opioid exposure history. Psychophar-macology 1994; 114:71-80.

63. Bickel WK, Stitzer ML, Liebson IA et al. Acute physical depen-dence in man: Effects of naloxone after brief morphine exposure. J Pharmacol Exp Ther 1988; 244:126-132.

64. Heishman SJ, Stitzer ML, Bigelow GE et al. Acute opioid physical dependence in postaddict humans: Naloxone dose effects after brief morphine exposure. J Pharmacol Exp Ther 1989; 248:127-134.

65. Heishman SJ, Stitzer ML, Bigelow GE et al. Acute opioid physical dependence in humans: Effect of varying the morphine-naloxone interval. J Pharmacol Exp Ther 1989; 250:485-491.

66. Heishman SJ, Stitzer ML, Bigelow GE et al. Acute opioid physical dependence in humans: Effect of naloxone at 6 and 24 hours postmorphine. Pharmacol Biochem Behav 1990; 36:393-399.

67. Jones RT. Dependence in non-addict humans after a single dose of morphine. In: Way EL, ed. Endogenous and Exogenous Opiate Agonists and Antagonists. New York: Pergamon Press, 1980: 557-560.

68. Kirby KC, Stitzer ML. Opioid physical dependence development in humans: Effect of time between agonist pretreatments. Psychop-harmacology 1993; 112:511-517.

69. Kirby KC, Stitzer ML, Heishman SJ. Acute opioid physical depen-dence in humans: Effect of varying the morphine-naloxone interval II. J Pharmacol Exp Ther 1990; 256:730-737.

70. Wright C, Bigelow GE, Stitzer ML et al. Acute physical depen-dence in humans: Repeated naloxone-precipitated withdrawal after a single dose of methadone. Drug Alcohol Depend 1991; 27:139-148.

71. Martin WR, Eades CG. A comparison between acute and chronic physical dependence in the chronic spinal dog. J Pharmacol Exp Ther 1964; 146:385-394.

72. Meyer DR, Sparber SB. Evidence of possible opiate dependence during the behavioral depressant action of a single dose of mor-phine. Life Sci 1977; 21:1087-1094.

73. White-Gbadebo D, Holtzman SG. Acute sensitization to opioid antagonists. Pharmacol Biochem Behav 1994; 474:559-566.

74. White-Gbadebo D, Holtzman SG. Naloxone pretreatment blocks acute morphine-induced sensitization. Psychopharmacology 1994; 114:225-228.

75. Cohen CA, Tonkiss J, Sparber SB. Acute opiate withdrawal in rats undernourished during infancy: Impact of the undernutrition method. Pharmacol Biochem Behav 1991; 39(2):329-335.

76. Cheney DL, Goldstein A. Tolerance to opioid narcotics: Time course and reversibility of physical dependence in mice. Nature 1971; 232:477-478.

77. Kosersky DS, Harris RA, Harris LS. Naloxone-precipitated jumping activity in mice following the acute administration of morphine. Eur J Pharmacol 1974; 26:122-124.

78. Krystal JH, Redmond DE Jr. A preliminary description of acute physical dependence on morphine in the vervet monkey. Pharmacol Biochem Behav 1983; 18:289-291.

79. Jacob JJ, Michaud GM. Acute physical dependence in the waking dog after a single low dose of morphine. Psychol Med 1974; 4:27-273.

80. Jacob JJ, Barthelemy CD, Tremblay EC et al. Potential usefulness of single-dose acute physical dependence on and tolerance to morphine for the evaluation of narcotic antagonists. In: Braude MC, Harris LS, May EL et al, eds. Narcotic Antagonists (Advances in Biochemical Psychopharmacology, Vol. 8). New York: Raven Press, 1974:299-318.

81. Ramabadran K. Naloxone-precipitated abstinence in mice, rats and gerbils acutely dependent on morphine. Life Sci 1983; 33(Suppl 1):385-388.

82. Smits SE. Quantitation of physical dependence in mice by naloxone-precipitated jumping after a single dose of morphine. Res Commun Chem Pathol Pharmacol 1995; 21:723.

83. Sofuoglu M, Sato J, Takemori AE. Maintenance of morphine dependence by naloxone in acutely dependent mice. J Pharmacol Exp Ther 1990; 254:841-846.

84. Wiley JN, Downs DA. Naloxone-precipitated jumping in mice pretreated with acute injections of opioids. Life Sci 1979; 25:797-802.

85. Schulteis G, Heyser CJ, Koob GF. Acute dependence on opiates: Progressive increase in severity with long intervals between successive morphine treatments. Soc Neurosci Abstr 1995; 21:723.

86. Adams JU, Holtzman SG. Pharmacologic characterization of the sensitization to the rate-decreasing effects of naltrexone induced by acute opioid pretreatment in rats. J Pharmacol Exp Ther 1990; 253:483-489.

87. Adams JU, Holtzman SG. Naltrexone-sensitizing effects of centrally administered morphine and opioid peptides. Eur J Pharmacol 1990; 193:67-73.

88. Easterling KW, Holtzman SG. Intracranial self-stimulation (ICSS): Sensitization to an opioid antagonist following chronic agonist pretreatment in rats. Soc Neurosci Abstr 1995; 21:721.

89. Young AM. Effects of acute morphine pretreatment on the rate-decreasing and antagonist activity of naloxone. Psychopharmacology 1986; 88:201-208.

90. Schaefer GJ, Michael RP. Changes in response rates and reinforcement thresholds for intracranial self-stimulation during morphine withdrawal. Pharmacol Biochem Behav 1986; 25:1263-1269.

91. Schulteis G, Markou A, Gold L et al. Relative sensitivity to naloxone of multiple indices of opiate withdrawal: A quantitative dose-response analysis. J Pharmacol Exp Ther 1994; 271:1391-1398.

92. Schwartz JM, Ksir C, Koob GF et al. Changes in locomotor response to beta-endorphin microinfusion during and after opiate abstinence syndrome—A proposal for a model of the onset of mania. Psychiatry Res 1982; 7:153-161.

93. Kalivas PW, Taylor S, Miller JS. Sensitization to repeated enkephalin administration into the ventral tegmental area of the rat: I. Behavioral characterization. J Pharmacol Exp Ther 1985; 235: 537-543.

94. Kalivas PW, Weber B. Amphetamine injection into the ventral mesencephalon sensitizes rats to peripheral amphetamine and cocaine. J Pharmacol Exp Ther 1988; 245:1095-1102.

95. Wise RA, Leeb K. Psychomotor-stimulant sensitization: A unitary phenomenon? Behav Pharmacol 1993; 4:339-349.

96. White FJ, Wolf ME. Psychomotor stimulants. In: Pratt JA, ed. The Biological Bases of Drug Tolerance and Dependence. London: Academic Press, 1991:153-197.

97. Henry DJ, White FJ. Repeated cocaine administration causes persistent enhancement of D1 dopamine receptor sensitivity within the rat nucleus accumbens. J Pharmacol Exp Ther 1991; 258: 882-889.

98. Ackerman JA, White FJ. A10 somatodendritic dopamine autoreceptor sensitivity following withdrawal from repeated cocaine treatment. Neurosci Lett 1990; 117:181-187.

99. Vezina P, Stewart J. The effect of dopamine receptor blockade on the development of sensitization to the locomotor activating effects of amphetamine and morphine. Brain Res 1989; 499:108-120.

100. Xu M, Hu XT, Cooper DC et al. Elimination of cocaine-induced hyperactivity and dopamine-mediated neurophysiological effects in dopamine D1 receptor mutant mice. Cell 1994; 79:945-955.

101. Dougherty GG, Ellinwood EH. Chronic d-amphetamine in the nucleus accumbens: Lack of tolerance or reverse tolerance of locomotor activity. Life Sci 1981; 28:2295-2298.
102. Criswell H, Mueller RA, Breese GR. Priming of D1 dopamine receptor responses; long-lasting behavioral supersensitivity to a D1-dopamine agonist following repeated administration to neonatal 6-OHDA-lesion rats. J Neurosci 1989; 9:125-133.
103. Koob GF, Cador M. Psychomotor stimulant sensitization: The corticotropin-releasing factor-steroid connection. Commentary on Wise and Leeb "Psychomotor-stimulant sensitization: A unitary phenomenon?". Behav Pharmacol 1993; 4:351-354.
104. Cole BJ, Cador M, Stinus L et al. Central administration of a CRF antagonist blocks the development of stress-induced behavioral sensitization. Brain Res 1990; 512:343-346.
105. Karler R, Calder LD, Turkanis SA. DNQX blockade of amphetamine behavioral sensitization. Brain Res 1991; 552:295-300.
106. Karler R, Calder LD, Chaudry IA et al. Blockade of "reverse tolerance" to cocaine and amphetamine by MK-801. Life Sci 1989; 45:599-606.
107. Karler R, Chaudry IA, Calder LD et al. Amphetamine behavioral sensitization and the excitatory amino acids. Brain Res 1990; 537:76-82.
108. Wolf ME, Khansa MR. Repeated administration of MK-801 produces sensitization to its own locomotor stimulant effects but blocks sensitization to amphetamine. Brain Res 1991; 562:164-168.
109. Stewart J, Druhan JP. Development of both conditioning and sensitization of the behavioral activating effects of amphetamine is blocked by the non-competitive NMDA receptor antagonist MK-801. Psychopharmacology 1993; 110:125-132.
110. Laulin JP, Larcher A, Bourguignon JJ et al. Hyperalgesia is a compensatory response associated with both acute and repeated heroin administration. XXVI International Narcotics Research Conference, University of St Andrews, Scotland 1995; 9-13 July 1995:70. (Abstract)

CHAPTER 7

TREATMENT OF OPIATE WITHDRAWAL

CLASSICAL COMPOUNDS USED FOR THE TREATMENT OF OPIATE WITHDRAWAL

There are a variety of procedures for opiate detoxification and treatment of opiate withdrawal, and these fall into two major classes: opiates and nonopiates. Opiates include the use of methadone, a long-acting oral analogue, and buprenorphine, a mixed agonist/antagonist. Nonopiates include clonidine (Catapres®).

Opiate withdrawal usually begins to be experienced by an addict 8-12 hours after their last injection of heroin (see chapter 1). Other opiates such as morphine (14-20 hours) or meperidine (4-6 hours) have a similar time course. An exception would be methadone-maintained individuals where the onset is delayed significantly (36-72 hours).

DETOXIFICATION WITH METHADONE

Methadone has a number of characteristics and advantages that make it useful in opiate detoxification.[1] Methadone has strong cross-dependence with other opiates, it is orally active, and it has a very long duration of action (24-36 hours). Also, by the oral route of administration methadone does not produce the pronounced highs associated with intravenous or smoked opiate use.

One of the first steps in methadone detoxification is to determine the degree of physical dependence in the opiate addict. Observation of measurable clinical signs is recommended,[1] and these include the following: increased heart rate (increase of 10 beats/ min), increased systolic blood pressure (10 mmHg over baseline), dilated pupils, and sweating. When all four signs are present, 10 mg of methadone is administered orally. Alternatively, rating scales have been used, and the dose of methadone given initially is graded by the severity of the withdrawal.

An evaluation should be repeated every 2-4 hours with methadone administered as often as necessary during the first 24 hours. Rarely, however, will a patient receive more than 40 mg of methadone. The exception would be a patient who is already maintained on high doses of methadone. The next day, the stabilizing dose, e.g., that given in the first 24 hours, should be given in divided doses. Beginning on the third day, the methadone dose is decreased by 5 mg/day until the patient is completely withdrawn.

The time course of methadone detoxification can range from 3-21 days using an outpatient procedure. Inpatient detoxification can usually be completed within 3-7 days but patients often prefer a more gradual reduction. All methadone should be dispensed in liquid form and consumed under direct supervision to avoid diversion of the drug to the street.[1]

BUPRENORPHINE IN OPIATE DETOXIFICATION

Buprenorphine is a partial opiate agonist (mixed agonist/antagonist) that is more potent than morphine as an analgesic.[2] It was introduced in England as an intramuscular analgesic in 1978 and in sublingual tablet form in 1981 where it has proved to be a safe, effective and long-lasting analgesic against moderate to severe pain.[3] It has a unique pharmacological profile of high affinity for opioid receptors, partial agonist activity at μ-receptors, κ-antagonist activity, a long duration of action, and slow elimination,[3] but at low doses (4 mg/day) it blocks withdrawal symptoms and at higher doses (8 mg/day) it can act as an opiate antagonist in the sense that it can precipitate opiate withdrawal.

Preliminary studies showed that 4 mg/day can block withdrawal symptoms in humans,[4] and subsequent studies have shown that for patients above daily methadone doses of 30 mg, it does not fully block withdrawal.[5] Buprenorphine produces a mild to moderate physical withdrawal syndrome in animal studies[3] and in humans, where studied.[6] To date, buprenorphine appears to have little physical dependence capacity[6] and low abuse potential.[7]

Buprenorphine use in opioid dependence treatment includes detoxification as well as maintenance.[5] The optimal maintenance dose appears to be 12-20 mg daily sublingual. For detoxification, a lower dose of 1-4 mg daily is preferred.

CLONIDINE IN OPIATE DETOXIFICATION

Clonidine (Catapres®) is a sympatholytic that is a nonopioid antihypertensive drug that has been known for some time to reduce the signs and symptoms of opiate withdrawal in animals.[8] Basically, clonidine has been used in three ways for opiate withdrawal: it has been used alone, in combination with methadone, or in combination with naloxone or naltrexone.[1,9-11]

For the use of clonidine alone, it is usually administered in a dose of 0.15-0.3 mg/day in three divided doses, not to exceed a daily dose of 1.2 mg.[11] After stabilization on clonidine for approximately 4 days, the drug dose is decreased and withdrawn over 4-6 days. The specific dose must be adjusted to reduce withdrawal symptoms as much as possible without causing hypotension. If a patient's blood pressure drops below 90/60 mmHg, then the drug is withheld. Detoxification from heroin can be completed in 5-10 days.[1]

For a combination of clonidine with methadone, 0.5-0.9 mg of clonidine was given per day with a gradual 5-10 mg drop per day in methadone.[9] Fifty percent of the subjects dropped to zero levels of methadone in 10 days.[9]

For a combination of clonidine with naltrexone, clonidine and naltrexone were administered in an inpatient study every 4 hours.[10] On days 1 and 2, the dose of clonidine was 0.4 mg, and the dose of naltrexone was 1 mg. On day 3, the dose of naltrexone was increased to 10 mg every 4 hours with clonidine administered three times daily only when needed. This procedure was repeated on day 4 but with a dose of 50 mg of naltrexone. Using this procedure, 38 out of 40 patients maintained on methadone completed treatment in 4-5 days and were discharged.

Several issues limit the usefulness of clonidine. Clonidine is contraindicated under certain medical conditions such as acute or chronic cardiac disorders, renal or metabolic diseases, and moderate to severe hypertension.[1] In outpatient settings there are problems with compliance, hypotension and overdoses. Inpatient procedures are safe and effective but expensive because of the need for up to 14 days of hospitalization.

NEW PERSPECTIVES: INHIBITORS OF THE ENKEPHALIN CATABOLISM

The endogenous enkephalins, like morphine and other opiates, interact in the central nervous system with the opioid receptors to produce their physiological and pharmacological responses. Increasing the level of endogenous opioid peptides by inhibiting the enzymes involved in their catabolism has been proposed as a means of inducing the pharmacological effects related to the activation of opioid receptors and minimizing the serious drawbacks produced by the acute as well as chronic administration of classical opiates.[12] Indeed, these side effects could be related to a ubiquitous overstimulation of opioid receptors in all brain areas containing opioid receptors, whereas the inhibitors of the enkephalin catabolism are expected to be active only in regions where enkephalins are either tonically or phasically released. Several pieces of evidence suggest that these inhibitors of the enkephalin-degrading enzymes may some day represent a promising therapeutic approach in analgesia and the management of addictive disorders.[13] Presented here are findings supporting this hypothesis and the new perspectives now available with the recent synthesis of mixed enkephalin-degrading enzyme inhibitors that are able to cross the blood-brain barrier and induce potent pharmacological responses after systemic administration.

PHYSIOLOGICAL DEGRADATION OF THE ENDOGENOUS ENKEPHALINS

The functional neurotransmission produced by neuropeptides such as the endogenous opioids is mainly interrupted by peptidases which cleave the biologically active peptide into inactive fragments, in contrast to the amine and amino acid transmitters which are mainly removed from the synaptic space by reuptake mechanisms, although such processes could also participate in the interruption of neuropeptide transmission.[14] Consistent with a neurotransmitter role, the endogenous enkephalins are quickly metabolized in the central nervous system, leading only to a weak and transient antinociception following intracerebroventricular administration of high doses of Met[5]-enkephalin (Tyr-Gly-Gly-Phe-Met) or Leu[5]-enkephalin (Tyr-Gly-Gly-Phe-Leu),[15] whereas a higher potency is obtained with enkephalin analogues protected from peptidase inactivation.[16,17]

Two different enzymes are involved in the physiological inactivation of the endogenous enkephalins. A first site of cleavage, in vivo, is the Gly[3]-Phe[4] bond which is hydrolyzed by a peptidase, originally designated enkephalinase[18] but since shown to be identical to the neutral metalloendopeptidase 24.11 (NEP) previously isolated from rabbit kidney.[19] A second enzyme, the aminopeptidase N (APN), is also responsible for the in vivo degradation of the enkephalins by cleavage of the Tyr[1]-Gly[2] bond.[20,21] NEP was found to be discretely distributed in rat brain, with a relatively good correspondence between the distribution of the enzyme, the opioid receptors[22] and the enkephalins.[23] The physiological relevance of NEP in enkephalin catabolism was firmly established by the naloxone-reversible antinociceptive properties elicited by the synthetic inhibitor thiorphan.[12] The distribution of APN is homogeneous in the brain, and no correlation with the localization of the endogenous enkephalins or opioid receptors was found by using immunohistochemistry techniques.[24] Interestingly, these two enzymes belong to the family of zinc metallopeptidases, therefore offering the possibility of designing mixed inhibitors (reviewed in Roques et al[25]).

DEVELOPMENT OF INHIBITORS
OF ENKEPHALIN-DEGRADING ENZYMES

Various specific inhibitors of NEP have been synthesized by using a model of the active site of metallopeptidases, deduced from the crystallographic analysis of the analogue enzyme thermolysin.[25,26] The introduction of strong metal-coordinating groups, such as thiol, carboxyl, phosphoryl or hydroxamate, on di- or tripeptide-like structures has led to obtaining different families of potent NEP inhibitors. The thiol-containing thiorphan was the first synthetic selective inhibitor of NEP.[12] Other thiol inhibitors were developed later, such as the retrothiorphan[27] and the phelorphan.[28] One of the inhibitors containing a phosphoryl group is phosphoramidon, a natural compound eliciting a potent inhibitory effect on NEP. The incorporation of a carboxyl group has been a strategy frequently used to obtain selective inhibitors of NEP[29] like SCH 39,370[30] and UK 69,578.[31] Selective inhibitors of NEP have also been developed as tritiaded probes, such as the hydroxamate derivate HACBO-Gly which has been widely used for autoradiographic studies.[21]

Various natural inhibitors of the aminopeptidases have been isolated from actinomycetes, such as the weakly active puromycin and the more potent peptide analogues bestatin and amastatin. However, these natural compounds have little selectivity for APN.[32] Synthetic inhibitors eliciting potent inhibitory properties and higher selectivity for APN have been designed. Thus, compounds that recognize the active site of APN and interact with the zinc atom, such as substituted aminoethane thiols, were found to be highly potent inhibitors of this enzyme.[33-35] Recently, carbaphethiol, a derivative of phenylalanine thiol protected by a hydrophobic carbamate group, has been reported to exhibit high inhibitory potency on APN after systemic administration,[36] but was found in vivo to be devoid of antinociceptive properties such as other APN inhibitors.[35,37]

The selective inhibitors of the NEP or APN have been shown to partially protect exogenous or endogenous opioid peptides in vitro by using slice preparations of brain[21,38,39] or spinal cord,[40] from which the enkephalins can be released by depolarization and the metabolites measured in the superfusion medium, or in vivo in anesthetized rats.[40] These inhibitors were reported to induce weak pharmacological responses caused by the protection of endogenous enkephalins from their catabolism.[41] They potentiate the antinociceptive responses of exogenously administered enkephalins or enkephalin analogues. However, the intrinsic naloxone-sensitive antinociceptive effects observed with the thiorphan prodrug acetorphan[41] have not been confirmed with these drugs.[37] This shows that when only one of the two enzymes implicated in the physiological degradation of the endogenous enkephalins is inhibited, the intrinsic pharmacological responses obtained are weak or even absent (reviewed in Roques et al[25]).

Therefore, taking into account the similarity in the active sites of NEP and APN, mixed inhibitors of both enzymes have been designed. This was first achieved using hydroxamate-containing inhibitors able to interact with the zinc atom of both enzymes. Kelatorphan was the first compound showing strong inhibitory effects on both NEP and APN activities.[42,43] As expected, mixed inhibitors produced stronger pharmacological responses than those obtained by inhibiting only one enzyme. Thus, kelatorphan decreased the dose of Met-enkephalin required to obtain 50% analgesia by a factor of 50,000 and induced intrinsic antinociceptive effects more potent than those observed after the association of the selective inhibitors bestatin and thiorphan.[42,43] Likewise, the amount of extracellular enkephalins in the spinally superfused rats was higher in the presence of kelatorphan than with the association of thiorphan and bestatin.[40] Using this concept of mixed inhibitors, a large number of analogues have been synthesized, all of them having a pseudodipeptide structure. For instance, RB 38A is another hydroxamate derivate as active as kelatorphan on NEP but three times more potent on APN.[44] This compound elicited stronger antinociceptive responses than kelatorphan and was the first inhibitor showing potent responses in all the various assays currently used to select analgesics, particularly on the tail-flick test in mice and rats.[45]

However, kelatorphan and its analogues have a high water solubility, which prevents them from crossing the blood-brain barrier. Efforts to improve their bioavailabilities have not been very successful, and therefore another strategy was employed consisting of linking highly potent thiol-containing APN and NEP inhibitors by a disulfide bond. In addition to the easy modulation of their hydrophilic properties, one of the main advantages of these mixed inhibitors is the stability of the disulfide bond in plasma. This is in contrast to its relatively rapid breakdown in the brain, allowing a predominant effect on the central nervous system.[46] It was demonstrated that these mixed inhibitors were able to cross the blood-brain barrier since after intravenous administration they displace the [3H]diprenorphine from its opioid binding sites in the mouse brain.[47] Among the different compounds synthesized, RB 101 was shown to be particularly active on different antinociceptive tests in rats and mice after systemic administration of relatively low doses[37] and to produce similar antidepressant-like effects on acute behavioral models.[48,49] Therefore, this compound allows one to investigate the pharmacological and therapeutic advantages that may result from replacing exogenous opiate administration with endogenous opioid augmentation by the protection of their endogenous enkephalins from their catabolism.

EFFECTS OF CHRONIC TREATMENT WITH INHIBITORS OF ENKEPHALIN-DEGRADING ENZYMES ON THE DEVELOPMENT OF OPIATE DEPENDENCE

Several studies have shown that the chronic administration of the inhibitors of the enkephalin catabolism produces fewer side effects than the chronic treatment with classical opiate agonists. Thus, the naloxone-precipitated withdrawal syndrome in rats has been investigated after central infusion into the lateral ventricle of comparable antinociceptive doses of the mixed inhibitor RB 38A, the selective NEP inhibitor RB 38B, the μ-selective agonist DAMGO, and the δ-selective agonist DSTBULET. DAMGO administration produced a severe physical dependence characterized by a high incidence of the different somatic signs of withdrawal after naloxone challenge. DSTBULET and RB 38A produced a moderate degree of dependence with a significant incidence of only two signs: wet dog shakes and changes in body temperature. No physical dependence was induced after chronic selective inhibition of NEP by RB 38B administration[50] (Fig. 7.1). In addition, chronic central infusion of DAMGO, DSTBULET and RB 38A produced a time-dependent reduction in their analgesic effects, and, after 120 hours of continuous infusion, only RB 38A was still able to induce significant antinociception.[50]

The results obtained with the mixed inhibitor RB 38A have been recently reinforced by experiments performed by systemic injection of RB 101. Thus, repeated administration of RB 101 in mice at a dose that produces a potent analgesic effect (160 mg/kg IP twice daily for 5 days)[37] did not induce tolerance to its antinociceptive response[51] and did not produce opioid dependence.[52]

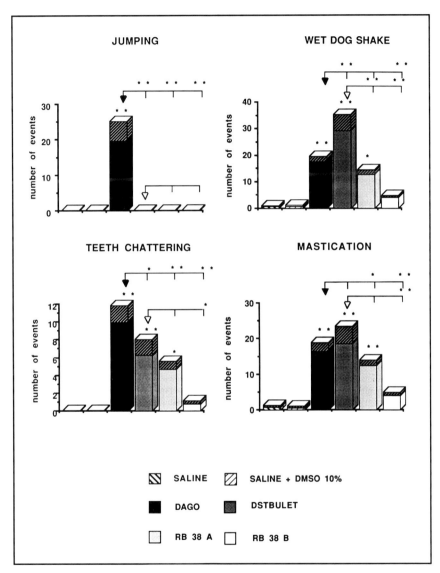

Fig. 7.1. Naloxone-precipitated withdrawal signs (jumping, wet dog shakes, teeth chattering and mastication) in rats chronically treated with DAMGO (0.18 µg/µl/h), DSTBULET (66.5 µg/µl/h), RB 38A (40 µg/µl/h), RB 38B (40 µg/µl/h) or control solutions (n = 10 per group). Values are mean ± SEM. *p<0.05; **p<0.01 vs control groups, when they are placed on the columns; or vs DSTBULET group, when they are placed on the opened arrow; or vs DAMGO group when they are placed on the closed arrow (Newman-Keuls test). Reproduced with permission from Maldonado R et al, Brain Res 1990; 520:247-254.

Under these experimental conditions, no somatic signs of withdrawal were observed when the animals were challenged with naloxone. Recent studies have also reported that the chronic administration of RB 101 in rats did not induce the development of tolerance at the peak effect time, although a slight decrease in the duration of the antinociceptive response was observed.[53]

The low degree of physical dependence produced after chronic administration of mixed enkephalin catabolism inhibitors is very likely due to a more selective stimulation of the opioid receptors by only the tonically released endogenous opioids, thus minimizing adaptive changes that usually occur after the general stimulation of opioid receptors by exogenously administered agonists.[25,54,55] The local concentration of the exogenously administered opioids probably largely exceeds the concentration of endogenous enkephalins in brain regions such as the periaqueductal gray matter and the locus coeruleus, which seem to play a crucial role in the development and expression of physical opiate dependence.[56,57]

EFFECTS OF THE INHIBITORS OF ENKEPHALIN-DEGRADING ENZYMES ON MORPHINE WITHDRAWAL SYNDROME

The exogenous administration of opioid peptides, such as β-endorphin,[58] dynorphin-(1-13)[59,60] and morphine-like pituitary peptides,[61] has been shown to reduce the severity of withdrawal syndrome in morphine-dependent animals and in heroin addicts. However, the enkephalins were relatively inefficient, probably as a consequence of their rapid degradation in vivo.[58] In agreement with this observation, the peptidase-resistant enkephalin analogues FK 33-824 and metkephamid completely suppress the behavioral expression of the opiate withdrawal syndrome in monkeys.[62]

When the activity of the endogenous opioid system was enhanced by inhibiting the enzymatic degradation of endogenous opioid peptides, an important decrease in the severity of opiate withdrawal was also observed. Thus, the nonspecific peptidase inhibitors apotropin and bacitracin[63] and the selective NEP inhibitors phosphoramidon,[64] thiorphan,[65] acetorphan[66] and SCH 34,828[67] minimized the severity of the naloxone-precipitated morphine withdrawal. However, the attenuating effect of these selective NEP inhibitors was limited since several signs remained unaffected, and in the case of acetorphan or SCH 34,828, some symptoms were even increased.[67] In agreement with the complementary role of NEP and APN in enkephalin inactivation, and with the results obtained in previous antinociceptive and behavioral studies, a greater inhibition of the withdrawal syndrome was induced by the administration of mixed inhibitors. Indeed, the effects of the central administration of the selective NEP inhibitor thiorphan and the mixed inhibitors kelatorphan and RB 38A were compared in the same model of naloxone-precipitated opiate withdrawal in rats[68] (Fig. 7.2). RB 38A and kelatorphan were more effective than thiorphan in decreasing most of the autonomic and behavioral signs of abstinence. The greater efficiency of the mixed inhibitors was very likely due to the resulting greater increase in enkephalins, especially in certain brain regions such as the caudal part of the periaqueductal gray matter which contains high levels of NEP[22] and is an important site of action for the expression of opiate withdrawal.[57,69] Accordingly, the local administration into the periaqueductal gray matter of selective or mixed inhibitors induced a reduction in the expression of withdrawal which was more intense and widespread than that observed after injection into the lateral ventricle.[56] Consequently, the attenuation of opiate withdrawal in these experiments seems to be related to the level of opioid receptor occupancy by exogenous or endogenous agonists in brain sites implicated in the manifestation of morphine abstinence.

The potential utilization of kelatorphan and its analogues in the clinical treatment of opiate addicts seems very unlikely since they are effective in suppressing opiate withdrawal in animal models but are unable to enter the brain following systemic administration. RB 101, the new mixed inhibitor able to induce potent antinociceptive responses after systemic administration,[37,46] represents a more promising approach. It has been recently reported that the systemic administration of RB 101 strongly attenuated the expression of naloxone-precipitated morphine withdrawal syndrome in rats.[70] This dose-dependent effect was observed at lower doses (5 mg/kg IV) than those reported to produce antinociceptive responses (10 mg/kg IV)[37,71] and reduced most of the withdrawal signs evaluated (8 of 14). Interestingly, a strong facilitation of RB 101 responses was observed when associated with the CCK-B

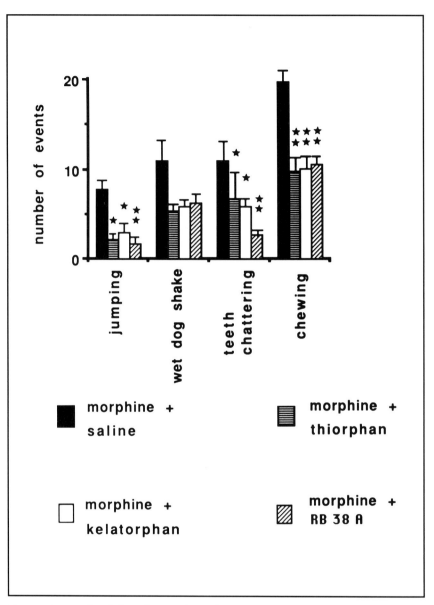

Fig. 7.2. Counted withdrawal signs after naloxone (5 mg/kg) in rats treated chronically with morphine: effect of pretreatment with saline (1 μl), thiorphan (20 μg/μl), kelatorphan (6.4 μg/μl) or RB 38A (2.4 μg/μl) into the lateral ventricle 15 minutes before naloxone. Values are mean ± SEM. Number of animals per group = 15. *p<0.05; **p<0.01: vs morphine + saline group (Mann-Whitney U test). Reproduced with permission from Maldonado R et al, Eur J Pharmacol 1989; 165:199-207.

antagonist PD-134,308. Indeed, this CCK compound did not modify the expression of morphine abstinence when given alone, but when co-administered with RB 101, strongly decreased the incidence of 12 of the 14 withdrawal signs measured[70] (Fig. 7.3). The facilitatory effect was particularly intense in peripherally mediated withdrawal signs such as salivation, lacrimation and rhinorhea.

A similar facilitatory effect was already reported for antinociceptive studies. PD-134,308 did not modify the antinociceptive threshold in rat tail-flick when given alone but strongly potentiated RB 101-induced antinociception.[53,72] PD-134,308, which has no affinity for opioid binding sites,[73] was found to facilitate the inhibition of the in vivo binding of [³H]diprenorphine induced by

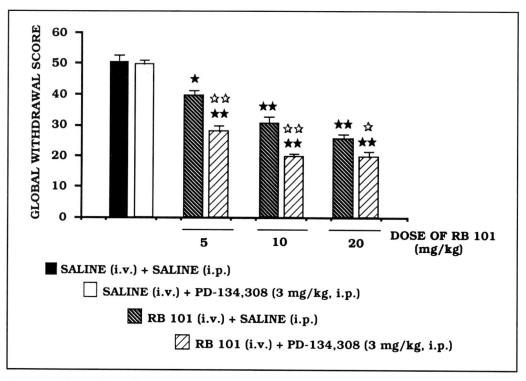

Fig. 7.3. Global withdrawal score after naloxone (1 mg/kg) in rats treated chronically with morphine: effect of pretreatment with saline, PD-134,308 (3 mg/kg IP), RB 101 (5, 10 and 20 mg/kg IV) or PD-134,308 (3 mg/kg IP) plus RB 101 (5, 10 and 20 mg/kg IV). Values are mean ±SEM. Number of animals per group = 10. *p<0.05; **p<0.01: vs saline + saline group; white stars vs RB 101 + saline group (Newman-Keuls test). Reproduced with permission from Maldonado R et al, Br J Pharmacol 1995; 114:1031-1039.

RB 101.[70] This result suggests that an increase in endogenous enkephalin levels induced by the CCK-B antagonist could participate in the facilitation of RB 101 behavioral responses. Accordingly, a modification in the release of β-endorphin after treatment
with CCK compounds has been previously reported,[74] and the activation of the endogenous opioid system can, in turn, regulate extracellular levels of CCK.[75] However, it would be difficult to explain the strong behavioral facilitation observed in these studies
only by considering an increase in endogenous enkephalin extracellular concentration because the magnitude of the facilitatory
response at the biochemical level was too small. Therefore, the
interaction between endogenous CCK and opioids could also be
due to direct or indirect changes in the μ-opioid receptor transduction processes. In agreement with this hypothesis, the modulation of endogenous opioid-induced antinociception by CCK seems
to be restricted to μ-opioid receptors since the enhanced
antinociceptive response obtained by the association of RB 101
and CCK-B antagonists was abolished by naloxone but not modified by the opioid δ-antagonist naltrindole.[71] These changes in the
transduction processes related to μ-opioid receptors could also participate in the facilitation observed in reducing morphine withdrawal response since μ-receptors are the most important in the
development and expression of physical opiate dependence[50,76,77]
(see chapter 5).

The ameliorative effects of the inhibitors of enkephalin catabolism have been reported in these studies on naloxone-precipitated
morphine withdrawal syndrome. However, in the clinical situation, opiate withdrawal is usually found when the addict cannot
obtain the abused compound, and not when an opiate antagonist
is administered. In order to more closely approach the human clinical condition, the effects of enkephalin catabolism inhibitors have
recently been investigated in an experimental model where a spontaneous morphine abstinence is induced by disrupting the opiate
agonist administration, and the evolution of withdrawal can be
examined under the influence of a substitute treatment.[78] The effects of RB 101, given alone or in association with the CCK-B
antagonist PD-134,308, were compared to those produced by some
compounds currently used to treat opiate dependence in humans,

such as clonidine and methadone. Methadone appeared to be the most effective compound in acutely decreasing spontaneous abstinence, but both methadone and RB 101 elicited the same effectiveness in reducing opiate withdrawal during the period of substitution treatment. This result suggests that RB 101 could represent an alternative to methadone in the maintenance of opiate addicts. The CCK-B antagonist did not show any effect when given alone and did not modify the responses induced by RB 101,[78] in contrast with the facilitatory effects obtained during naloxone-precipitated morphine withdrawal.[70] Consequently, it could be possible that the acute administration of the opiate antagonist could immediately induce a phasic release of endogenous CCK that would participate in the expression of naloxone-precipitated morphine withdrawal. In this case, the administration of a CCK-B antagonist would be able to antagonize the effect of endogenous CCK, and to potentiate the antiwithdrawal responses of the enkephalin catabolism inhibitor. On the other hand, this phasic release of CCK would not appear during spontaneous abstinence, and the CCK-B antagonist would therefore be unable to potentiate the response of RB 101.[78]

Considering the weak opiate-like side effects observed after chronic treatment with the peptidase inhibitors such as RB 101,[25] one can speculate that induction of enkephalinergic system activation by means of potent inhibitors of enkephalin catabolism able to cross the blood-brain barrier may play a therapeutic role in the treatment of opiate dependence. Consistent with this hypothesis, clinical studies have already been performed with the selective NEP inhibitor acetorphan. The effects of acetorphan were compared in a double-blind trial with those of clonidine for the treatment of the opiate withdrawal syndrome. Acetorphan induced a more marked effect on several objective signs than did clonidine, whereas the two drugs exhibited similar efficacy on the subjective components of withdrawal.[79] Taking into account that the pharmacological responses of the selective inhibitors of NEP, such as acetorphan, are very weak in comparison to those induced by the mixed inhibitors,[25,37] the opportunity to use RB 101 by a peripheral route represents an important step toward the development of new therapeutic tools, allowing one to replace the exogenous opiates by their endogenous analogues. Therefore, this mixed inhibitor, given alone or co-administered with CCK-B antagonists, has a promising potential role in the management of opiate withdrawal syndrome in humans.

NEW PERSPECTIVES:
TRANSCUTANEOUS ELECTRICAL STIMULATION

Since the discovery of electricity, there have been numerous attempts to produce sleep and general anesthesia by means of electrical stimulation applied through the brain with transcranial electrodes. In most of these studies, low-frequency currents were used, and in spite of positive results, the current application could not be applied for more than half an hour, and the intensity could not be raised without producing serious side effects and discomfort.[11,80-85]

A new step forward was made by the introduction of a special form of transcutaneous cranial electrical stimulation (TCES) using a complex high-frequency (HF) waveform derived from a mathematical analysis of the electrical characteristics of the biological tissue (Fig. 7.4).

TCES consists of a high-frequency, intermittent, balanced current which facilitates the penetration of electric fields throughout the brain tissue, with no modification of the tissue conductivity.[86-89] TCES is asymptomatic, and the intensity of the current can be raised up to 100-200 mA, peak to peak, without inducing any unpleasant sensations, cutaneous damage (burns), muscular contractures or other serious side effects, even when applied continuously for hours or days. Several studies have demonstrated that this method is very effective for potentiation of anesthetic effects in urologic, thoracic, gastrointestinal, orthopedic and gynecologic surgeries.[90-95] It was shown that TCES increased N_2O anesthetic potency, allowed a reduction of the need for opiate analgesics, and induced a better quality of anesthesia followed by a long-lasting postoperative analgesic period.[96,97] TCES was then tested on opiate addicts during withdrawal because it was hypothesized that TCES increased release of endogenous opioid peptides with no side effects ever being reported. Results were spectacular—TCES attenuated acute withdrawal symptoms during opiate detoxifica-

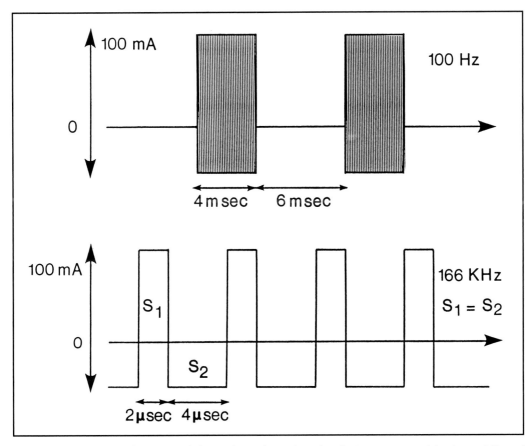

Fig. 7.4. Characteristics of transcranial electrical stimulation (TCES) with Limoge current. Stimulators delivered a high-frequency (HF = 166 kHz, 2 μsec+, 4 μsec-, with an exponential ascent and acute fall signal), intermittent low-frequency (LF = 100 Hz, 4 msec) balanced current (S1 = S2). Reproduced with permission from Stinus L et al, Pain 1990; 42:351-363.

tion. The clinical efficacy of this treatment was confirmed by a double-blind study.[98,99]

However, most human studies published in the 1970s suffer from lack of rigorous controls. In the last few years using animal models and rigorous blind schedules, it has been shown that TCES, which, per se, does not alter pain sensitivity in control rats, was able to potentiate opiate-induced analgesia when the drug was administered peripherally or centrally[100,101] (Fig. 7.5).

Moreover, TCES was able to reduce spontaneously-induced withdrawal syndrome in morphine-dependent rats, while the intensity of naloxone-precipitated withdrawal was unchanged by

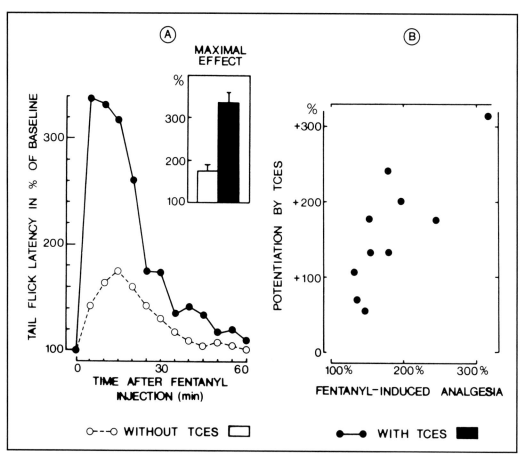

Fig. 7.5. Potentiation of morphine-induced analgesia by transcutaneous electrical stimulation (TCES) application. Blind experiments testing the effects of TCES on morphine-induced analgesia (10 mg/kg SC). Rats were tested twice, randomly with or without TCES, at 2-week intervals. Pain sensitivity was evaluated by the measurement of tail-flick latency (water bath 52%C). Stimulation (100 mA, peak to peak, frontal electrode connected to the negative pole, retromastoid electrodes connected to the positive pole) started 3 hours before the drug injection. Left panel: tail-flick latency (in % of baseline) at various times after drug injection. Right panel: maximal individual increase in tail-flick latency after drug injection and maximal individual potentiation of analgesic effects induced by TCES. Reproduced with permission from Stinus L et al, Pain 1990; 42:351-363.

TCES[101] (Fig. 7.6). These results suggested, indirectly, the involvement of endogenous opioid peptides in TCES-induced attenuation of spontaneous opiate withdrawal. This hypothesis was confirmed by other data which showed that TCES potentiated halothane-induced anesthesia and that this potentiation was completely inhibited by naloxone and increased by thiorphan, an inhibitor of enkephalin-degrading enzymes.[102] More recent data in-

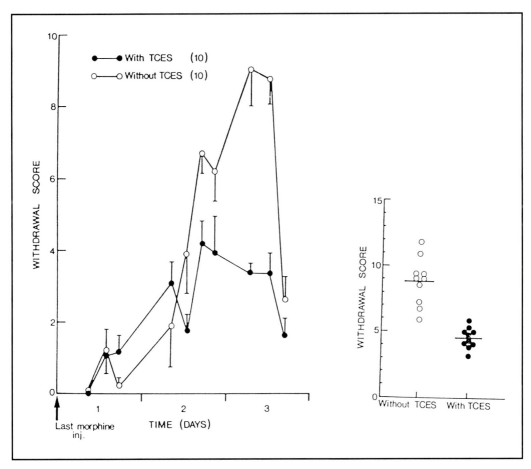

Fig. 7.6. Continuous application of transcranial electrical stimulation (TCES) with Limoge current attenuates spontaneously induced opiate withdrawal. Opiate dependence was induced by chronic morphine treatment in which rats received increasing doses of morphine (up to 90 mg/kg ip) twice a day for 10 days. TCES (100 mA, peak to peak) started 3 hours after the last injection of morphine and was continuously applied during the course of the experiment (3 days). Left panel: Overall results; withdrawal was scored by Gellert-Holtzman's scale. Mean scores over the 3 days of testing were 2.52 for the experimental group (with TCES) and 4.64 for controls (without TCES) (p<0.0001). Right panel: Individual results computed as the mean of the three highest scores obtained during the 3 days: experimental group (with TCES) 4.53, controls (without TCES) 8.78 (p<0.0001). (From Auriacombe et al.[101])

dicate that TCES potentiates droperidol- and diazepam-induced inhibition of dorsal immobility response and that a 3 hour TCES session increases the locomotor activity of rats introduced to a novel environment, while TCES was without effect after habituation to the testing chambers. Finally, while the amount of food and water intake was not altered by TCES, eating patterns were modified. Stimulated rats ate fewer meals which were of longer duration and switched less from one biscuit to another, indicating perhaps an anxiolytic effect of TCES which should be explored further.[101]

TCES, then, with Limoge current, from both animal and human studies, appears to be a safe procedure applicable continuously in humans for several days with no risk of overdose or abuse. The clinical schedule generally used to alleviate withdrawal symptomatology in opiate addicts lasts 10 days. TCES is delivered through three silver patch electrodes. One electrode is connected to the negative pole of the stimulator and is located on the metopic suture just above the nose; two posterior electrodes which are connected to the positive pole of the stimulator are located in the retromastoideum position. The intensity of TCES is adjusted to obtain 250-300 mA, peak to peak. As already indicated, TCES is asymptomatic. During the first 4 days of abstinence patients received TCES on a continuous basis, then intermittently according to the patient's comfort for the next 6 days.

REFERENCES

1. Gelenberg AJ, Bassuk EL, Schoonover SC. The Practitioner's Guide to Psychoactive Drugs. 3rd ed. New York: Plenum Publishing Corp., 1991.
2. Cowan A, Doxey JC, Harry EJR. The animal pharmacology of buprenorphine, an oripavine analgesic agent. Br J Pharmacol 1977; 69:547-554.
3. Cowan A. Update on the general pharmacology of buprenorphine. In: Buprenorphine: Combatting Drug Abuse with a Unique Opioid. Wiley-Liss, Inc., 1995:31-47.
4. Kosten TR, Kleber HD. Buprenorphine detoxification from opioid dependence: A pilot study. Life Sci 1988; 42:635-641.
5. Cowan A, Lewis JW. Buprenorphine: Combatting Drug Abuse with a Unique Opioid. New York: Wiley Liss, 1995.
6. Fudala PJ, Jaffe JH, Dax EM et al. Use of buprenorphine in the treatment of opioid addiction. II. Physiologic and behavioral effects of daily and alternate-day administration and abrupt withdrawal. Clin Pharmacol Ther 1990; 47:525-534.
7. Lewis JW, Rance MJ, Sanger DJ. The pharmacology and abuse potential of buprenorphine: A new antagonist and analgesic. In: Mello NK, ed. Advances in Substance Abuse—Behavioral and Biological Research (Vol. 3). Greenwich, CT: JAI Press, 1983:103-154.
8. Tseng LF, Loh HH, Wei ET. Effects of clonidine on morphine withdrawal signs in the rat. Eur J Pharmacol 1975; 30:93-99.

9. Washton AM, Resnick RB. Outpatient opiate detoxification with clonidine. J Clin Psychiatry 1982; 43:39-41.

10. Charney DS, Heninger GR, Kleber HD. The combined use of clonidine and naltrexone as a rapid, safe and effective treatment of abrupt withdrawal from methadone. Am J Psychiatry 1986; 143:831-837.

11. Traub SL. Clonidine for opiate withdrawal. Hospital Formulations 1985; 20:77-80.

12. Roques BP, Fournié-Zaluski MC, Soroca E et al. The enkephalinase inhibitor thiorphan shows antinociceptive activity in mice. Nature 1980; 288:286-288.

13. Roques BP, Noble F. Dual inhibitors of enkephalin-degrading enzymes (neutral endopeptidase 24.11 and aminopeptidase N) as potential new medications in the management of pain and opioid addiction. NIDA Technical Review on Discovery of Novel Opioid Medications, RS Rapaka and H Sorer (eds), 1995; 147:104-145.

14. Migaud M, Roques BP, Durieux C. Evidence for a high-affinity uptake system for cholecystokinin octapeptide (CCK-8) in rat cortical synaptosomes. Eur J Neurosci 1995; 7:1074-1079.

15. Belluzi JD, Grant N, Garsky V et al. Analgesia induced in vivo by central administration of enkephalin in rat. Nature 1976; 260:625-626.

16. Pert C, Pert A, Chang JK et al. [D-Ala^2]-Met-enkephalinamide: A potent, long-lasting synthetic pentapeptide analgesic. Science 1976; 194:330-332.

17. Fournié-Zaluski MC, Perdrisot R, Gacel G et al. Inhibitory potency of various peptides on enkephalinase activity from mouse striatum. Biochem Biophys Res Commun 1979; 91:130-135.

18. Malfroy B, Swerts JP, Guyon A et al. High-affinity enkephalin-degrading peptidase in mouse brain and its enhanced activity following morphine. Nature 1978; 276:523-526.

19. Kerr MA, Kenny AJ. The molecular weight and properties of a neutral metallo-endopeptidase from rabbit kidney brush border. Biochem J 1974; 137:489-495.

20. Hambrook JM, Morgan BA, Rance MJ et al. Mode of deactivation of the enkephalins by rat and human plasma and rat brain homogenates. Nature 1976; 262:782-783.

21. Waksman G, Bouboutou R, Devin J et al. In vitro and in vivo effects of kelatorphan on enkephalin metabolism in rodent brain. Eur J Pharmacol 1985; 117:233-243.

22. Waksman G, Hamel E, Fournié-Zaluski MC et al. Autoradiographic comparison of the distribution of the neutral endopeptidase "enkephalinase" and of mu and delta opioid receptors in rat brain. Proc Natl Acad Sci USA 1986; 83:1523-1527.

23. Pollard M, Bouthenet ML, Moreau J et al. Detailed immuno-autoradiographic mapping system comparison with enkephalins and SP. Neuroscience 1989; 30:339-376.

24. Gros C, Solhonne B, Pollard H et al. Immunohistochemical and subcellular studies of aminopeptidase M localization in rat brain: Microvessels and synaptic membranes. In: Holaday JW, Law P-Y, Herz A, eds. Progress in Opioid Research. Rockville: NIDA Research Monograph, DHHS, 1986:75:303-306.

25. Roques BP, Noble F, Daugé V et al. Neutral endopeptidase 24.11: Structure, inhibition, and experimental and clinical pharmacology. Pharmacol Rev 1993; 45:87-146.

26. Fournié-Zaluski MC. Design and evaluation of inhibitors of enkephalin-degrading enzymes. Neurochem Int 1988; 12:375-382.

27. Roques BP, Lucas-Soroca E, Chaillet P et al. Complete differentiation between "enkephalinase" and angiotensin coverting enzyme inhibition by retro-thiorphan. Proc Natl Acad Sci USA 1983; 80:3178-3182.

28. Van Amsterdan JGC, Van Buren KJM, Blod MWH et al. Synthesis of enkephalinase B inhibitors and their activity on isolated enkephalin-degrading enzymes. Eur J Pharmacol 1987; 135:411-418.

29. Fournié-Zaluski MC, Chaillet P, Soroca-Lucas E et al. New carboxyalkyl inhibitors of brain enkephalinase: Synthesis, biological activity, and analgesic properties. J Med Chem 1983; 26:60-65.

30. Sybertz EJ, Chiu PJS, Vemulapalli S et al. SCH 39370, a neutral metalloendopeptidase inhibitor, potentiates biological responses of atrial natriuretic factor and lowers blood pressure in deoxycorticosterone acetate-sodium hypertensive rats. J Pharmacol Exp Ther 1989; 250:624-631.

31. Northridge DB, Alabaster CT, Connell JMC et al. Effects of UK 69578: A novel atriopeptidase inhibitor. Lancet 1989; 2:591-593.

32. Rich DH. Peptidase inhibitors. In: Sammes PG, Taylor JB, eds. Comprehensive Medicinal Chemistry. The Rational Design, Mechanistic Study and Therapeutic Application of Chemical Compounds, Vol. 2. Oxford: Pergamon, 1990:391-441.

33. Chan WWC. L-leucinethiol, a potent inhibitor of leucine aminopeptidase. Biochem Biophys Res Commun 1983; 116:297-302.

34. Roques BP. Physiological role of endogenous peptide effectors studied with peptidase inhibitors. Kidney Int 1988; 34:S27-S33.

35. Fournié-Zaluski MC, Coric P, Turcaud S et al. Potent and systemically active aminopeptidase N inhibitors designed from active-site investigation. J Med Chem 1992; 35:1259-1266.

36. Gros C, Giros B, Schwartz JC et al. Potent inhibition of cerebral aminopeptidases by carbaphethiol, a parenterally active compound. Neuropeptides 1988; 12:111-118.

37. Noble F, Soleihac JM, Soroca-Lucas E et al. Inhibition of the enkephalin-metabolizing enzymes by the first systemically active mixed inhibitor prodrug RB 101 induces potent analgesic responses in mice and rats. J Pharmacol Exp Ther 1992; 261:181-190.

38. Patey G, De La Baume S, Schwartz JC et al. Selective protection of methionine enkephalin released from brain slices by thiorphan, a potent enkephalinase inhibitor. Science 1981; 212:1153-1155.

39. Alstein M, Bacher E, Vogel Z et al. Protection of enkephalins from enzymatic degradation utilizing selective metal-chelating inhibitors. Eur J Pharmacol 1983; 91:353-361.

40. Bourgoin S, Le Bars D, Artaud F et al. Effects of kelatorphan and other peptidase inhibitors on the in vitro and in vivo release of methionine-enkephalin-like material from the rat spinal cord. J Pharmacol Exp Ther 1986; 238:360-366.

41. Lecomte JM, Costentin J, Vlaiculescu A et al. Pharmacological properties of acetorphan, a parenterally active enkephalinase inhibitor. J Pharmacol Exp Ther 1986; 237:937-944.

42. Fournié-Zaluski MC, Chaillet P, Bouboutou R et al. Analgesic effects of kelatorphan, a new highly potent inhibitor of multiple enkephalin-degrading enzymes. Eur J Pharmacol 1984; 102:525-528.

43. Fournié-Zaluski MC, Coulaud A, Bouboutou R et al. New bidentates as full inhibitors of enkephalin-degrading enzymes: Synthesis and analgesic properties. J Med Chem 1985; 28:1158-1169.

44. Xie J, Soleilhac JM, Schmidt C et al. New kelatorphan-related inhibitors of enkephalin metabolism improved antinociceptive properties. J Med Chem 1989; 32:1497-1503.

45. Schmidt C, Peyroux J, Noble F et al. Analgesic responses elicited by endogenous enkephalins (protected by mixed peptidase inhibitors) in a variety of morphine-sensitive noxious tests. Eur J Pharmacol 1991; 192:253-262.

46. Fournié-Zaluski MC, Coric P, Turcaud S et al. "Mixed inhibitor-Prodrug" as a new approach toward systemically active inhibitors of enkephalin-degrading enzymes. J Med Chem 1992; 35: 2473-2481.

47. Ruiz-Gayo M, Baamonde A, Turcaud S et al. In vivo occupation of mouse brain opioid receptors by endogenous enkephalins: Blockade of enkephalin-degrading enzymes by RB 101 inhibits [3H] diprenorphine binding. Brain Res 1992; 571:306-312.

48. Baamonde A, Daugé V, Ruiz-Gayo M et al. Antidepressant-type effects of endogenous enkephalins protected by systemic RB 101 are mediated by opioid delta and dopamine D1 receptor stimulation. Eur J Pharmacol 1992; 216:157-166.

49. Smadja C, Maldonado R, Turcaud S et al. Opposite role of CCK-A and CCK-B receptors in the modulation of endogenous enkepha-

lins' antidepressant-like effects. Psychopharmacology 1995; 120:400-408.

50. Maldonado R, Feger J, Fournié-Zaluski MC et al. Differences in physical dependence induced by selective mu or delta opioid agonists and by endogenous enkephalins protected by peptidase inhibitors. Brain Res 1990; 520:247-254.

51. Noble F, Coric P, Fournié-Zaluski MC et al. Lack of physical dependence in mice after repeated systemic administration of the mixed inhibitor prodrug of enkephalin-degrading enzymes RB 101. Eur J Pharmacol 1992; 223:91-96.

52. Noble F, Turcaud S, Fournié-Zaluski MC et al. Repeated systemic administration of the mixed inhibitor of enkephalin-degrading enzyme, RB 101, does not induce either antinociceptive tolerance or cross-tolerance with morphine. Eur J Pharmacol 1992; 223:83-89.

53. Valverde O, Blommaert A, Turcaud S et al. The CCK-B antagonist PD-134,308 induces a long-lasting potentiation of antinociceptive responses mediated by endogenous enkaphalins in the rat tail-flick test. Eur J Pharmacol 1995; 286:79-93.

54. Williams JT, Christie MJ, North RA et al. Potentiation of enkephalin action by peptidase inhibitors in rat locus coeruleus in vitro. J Pharmacol Exp Ther 1987; 243:397-401.

55. De Witte PH, Heidbreder CH, Roques BP. Kelatorphan, a potent enkephalinase inhibitor, and opioid receptor agonists DAGO and DTLET differentially modulate self-stimulation behavior depending on the site of administration. Neuropharmacology 1989; 28:667-676.

56. Maldonado R, Fournié-Zaluski MC, Roques BP. Attenuation of the morphine withdrawal syndrome by inhibition of the endogenous enkephalin catabolism into the periaqueductal gray matter. Naunyn Schmiedebergs Arch Pharmacol 1992; 345:466-472.

57. Bozarth MA. Physical dependence produced by central morphine infusions: An anatomical mapping study. Neurosci Biobehav Rev 1994; 18:373-383.

58. Tseng LF, Loh HH, Li CH. β-endorphin: Cross-tolerance to and cross-physical dependence on morphine. Proc Natl Acad Sci USA 1976; 73:4187-4189.

59. Wen HL, Ho WKK. Suppression of withdrawal symptoms by dynorphin in heroin addicts. Eur J Pharmacol 1982; 82:183-186.

60. Wen HL, Ho WKK, Wen PYC. Comparison of the effectiveness of different opioid peptides in suppressing heroin withdrawal. Eur J Pharmacol 1984; 100:155-163.

61. Bläsig J, Herz A. Tolerance and dependence induced by morphine-like pituitary peptides in rat. Naunyn Schmiedebergs Arch Pharmacol 1976; 294:297-300.

62. Gmerek DE, Katz JL, France CP et al. Systemic and intracerebro-ventricular effects of opioid peptides in withdrawn morphine-dependent rhesus monkeys. Life Sci 1983; 33(Suppl. I):361-369.

63. Pinsky C, Dua AK, Labella FS. Peptidase inhibitors reduce opiate narcotic withdrawal signs, including seizure activity, in rats. Brain Res 1982; 243:301-307.

64. Dzoljic MR, Rademaker B, Poel-Heisterkamp AL et al. Enkephalinase inhibition suppresses naloxone-induced jumpint in morphine-dependent mice. Arch Int Pharmacodyn Ther 1986; 283:222-228.

65. Haffmans J, Dzoljic MR. Inhibition of enkephalinase activity attenuates naloxone-precipitated withdrawal symptoms. Gen Pharmacol 1987; 18:103-105.

66. Livingston SJ, Sewell RDE, Rooney KF et al. Amelioration of naloxone-precipitated opioid withdrawal symptoms by peripheral administration of the enkephalinase inhibitor acetorphan. Psychopharmacology 1988; 94:540-544.

67. Dzoljic MR, Bokszanska A, Korenhof AM et al. The effects of orally active enkephalinase inhibitors on morphine withdrawal syndrome. NeuroReport 1992; 3:637-640.

68. Maldonado R, Daugé V, Callebert J et al. Comparison of selective and complete inhibitors of enkephalin-degrading enzymes on morphine withdrawal syndrome. Eur J Pharmacol 1989; 165:199-207.

69. Maldonado R, Stinus L, Gold LH et al. Role of different brain structures in the expression of the physical morphine withdrawal syndrome. J Pharmacol Exp Ther 1992; 261:669-677.

70. Maldonado R, Valverde O, Ducos B et al. Inhibition of morphine withdrawal syndrome by the association of a peptidase inhibitor and a CCK-B antagonist. Br J Pharmacol 1995; 114:1031-1039.

71. Maldonado R, Derrien M, Noble F et al. Association of a peptidase inhibitor and a CCK-B antagonist strongly potentiates antinociception mediated by endogenous enkephalins. NeuroReport 1993; 7:947-950.

72. Valverde O, Maldonado R, Fournié-Zaluski MC et al. CCK-B antagonists strongly potentiate antinociception mediated by endogenous enkephalins. J Pharmacol Exp Ther 1994; 270:77-88.

73. Hughes J, Boden P, Costall B et al. Development of a class of selective cholecystokinin type B receptor antagonists having potent anxiolytic activity. Proc Natl Acad Sci USA 1990; 87:6728-6732.

74. Millington WR, Mueller GP, Lavigne GJ. Cholecystokinin type A and type B receptor antagonists produce opposing effects on cholecystokinin-stimulated beta-endorphin secretion from the rat pituitary. J Pharmacol Exp Ther 1992; 261:454-461.

75. Ruiz-Gayo M, Durieux C, Fournié-Zaluski MC et al. Stimulation of delta opioid receptors reduces the in vivo binding of the

CCK-B-selective agonist [³H]pBC 264: Evidence for a physiological regulation of CCKergic systems by endogenous enkephalins. J Neurochem 1992; 59:1805-1811.

76. Cowan A, Zhu XZ, Mosberg HI et al. Direct dependence studies in rats with agents selective for different types of opioid receptor. J Pharmacol Exp Ther 1988; 246:950-955.

77. Maldonado R, Negus S, Koob GF. Precipitation of morphine withdrawal syndrome in rats by administration of mu-, delta- and kappa-selective opioid antagonists. Neuropharmacology 1992; 31: 1231-1241.

78. Ruiz F, Fournié-Zaluski MC, Roques BP et al. The inhibitor of enkephalin catabolism, RB 101, induces a similar decrease in spontaneous morphine abstinence syndrome than methadone; First European Congress of Pharmacology, Milan. Pharmacol Res 1995; 31(Suppl):113.

79. Hartmann F, Poirier MF, Bourdel MC et al. Comparison of acetorphan with clonidine for opiate withdrawal symptoms. Am J Psychiatry 1991; 148:627-629.

80. Hardy JD, Fabian LW, Turner MD. Electrical anesthesia for major surgery. JAMA 1961; 175:599-601.

81. Smith RH, Goodwin G, Fowler E et al. Electronarcosis produced by a combination of direct and alternate current. A preliminary study: 1. Apparatus and electrodes. Anesthesiology 1961; 22: 163-166.

82. Smith RH. Electrical Anesthesia. Springfield: C.C.Thomas, 1963.

83. Smith RH. Electroanesthesia. Anesth Analg 1971; 34:60-72.

84. Herin RA. Electroanesthesia: A review of the literature (1819-1965). Activ Nerv Super 1968; 10:439-454.

85. Kuzin MI, Satchov VI. Some results of fifteen years of electroanesthesia research in surgical clinic and experiment. In: Limoge A, Cara M, Debras C, eds. Electrotherapeutic Sleep and Electroanesthesia. Paris: Masson, 1978:93-95.

86. Limoge A. In: Johnson RM, ed. An Introduction to Electroanesthesia. Baltimore: University Park Press, 1975:1-121.

87. Limoge A, Boisgontier MT. Characteristic of electric currents used in human anesthesiology. In: Ribak B, ed. Advanced Technology. Germantown, PA: Sythoff and Noordhoff, 1979:437-446.

88. Limoge A, Louville Y, Barritault L et al. Electrical anesthesia. In: Spierdijk J, Feldman SA, Mattie H et al, eds. Developments in Drugs Used in Anesthesia. Boston: Leiden University Press, 1981:121-134.

89. Prieur G, Dubois F, Barritault L et al. Approche mathématique de l'action biologique des courants de Limoge. J Biophysique Mécanique 1985; 9:67-74.

90. Cara M, Cara-Beurton M, Debras C et al. Essais d'anesthésie électrique chez l'homme. Ann Anesth Franç 1972; 13:521-526.

91. Kucera H, Kubista E, Haghghi B et al. The effects of electroanalgesia in obstetrics (technique by Limoge). In: Limoge A, Cara M, Debras C, eds. Electrotherapeutic Sleep and Electroanesthesia. Paris: Masson, 1978:73-77.

92. Bourdallé-Badie C, Gardien P, Laforge E et al. Les anesthésies de longue durée. Anesth Annual Réan 1980; 37:523-526.

93. Champagne C, Papiernik E, Therry JP et al. Electrostimulation cérébrale transcutanée pour les courants de Limoge au cours de l'accouchement. Ann Fr Anesth 1984; 3:405-413.

94. Coeytaux R, Atinault A, Cazalaa JB et al. Etude à double insu de l'efficacité de l'anesthésie électromédicamenteuse: A propos de 50 adénomectomies prostatiques. Agressologie 1977; 18:213-215.

95. Vigreux G, Onimus R, Linoge A et al. Utilisation clinique des courants impulsionnels de haute fréquence en anesthésie générale chez l'homme. Ann Anesth Franç 1978; 19:455-482.

96. Stanley TH, Cazalaa JA, Atinault A et al. Transcutaneous cranial electrical stimulation decreases narcotic requirements during neuroleptic anesthesia and operation in man. Anesth Analg 1982; 61:863-866.

97. Stanley TH, Cazalaa JA, Limoge A et al. Transcutaneous cranial electrical stimulation increases the potency of nitrous oxide in humans. Anesthesiology 1982; 57:293-297.

98. Daulouéde JP, Daubech JF, Bourdallé-Badie C et al. Une nouvelle méthode de sevrage des toxicomanes par utilisation du courant de Limoge. Ann Med Psychol 1980; 138:359-370.

99. Ellison F, Ellison W, Daulouéde JP et al. Opiate withdrawal and electrostimulation double-blind experiments. Encéphale 1987; 13:225-229.

100. Stinus L, Auriacombe M, Tignol J et al. Transcranial electrical stimulation with high frequency intermittent current (Limoge's) potentiates opiate-induced analgesia. Pain 1990; 42:351-363.

101. Auriacombe M, Tignol J, Le Moal M et al. Transcutaneous electrical stimulation with limoge current potentiates morphine analgesia and attenuates opiate abstinence syndrome. Biol Psychiatry 1990; 28:650-656.

102. Mantz J, Azerad J, Limoge A et al. Transcranial electrical stimulation with Limoge's current decreases halothane requirements in rats. Anesthesiology 1992; 76:253-260.

CHAPTER 8

THE ROLE OF OPIATE WITHDRAWAL IN ADDICTION

The role of withdrawal in drug addiction has diminished in recent years as much research has shown the powerful effects of opiates to produce positive reinforcement. A major impetus for this conceptual framework was the observation that animals and humans could take opiates under limited access situations without any evidence of physical dependence.[1] This view of a more limited role of withdrawal in addiction is reflected in the change of withdrawal being only one of seven criteria for a definition of addiction in DSM-IV[2] rather than being an essential criteria for addiction.[3]

However, recent considerations of the withdrawal in opiate addiction[4] have made a major distinction between physical and motivational aspects of withdrawal, and this separation forces the reevaluation of the role of withdrawal addiction. An important factor supporting an important role of motivational aspects of withdrawal in addiction is the success of methadone maintenance which will be described below. In addition, the experimental demonstration of long-lasting neurobiological perturbations in the brain reward circuits at every level of analysis—system, cellular and molecular—provides strong empirical support for neuroadaptation hypotheses and for future interventions during abstinence and protracted abstinence.

PROGRAMS OF METHADONE MAINTENANCE

Methadone maintenance has a theoretical basis in the observation that chronic opioid use induces long-lasting, perhaps even permanent, physiological changes that result in a strong motivation to take the drug, and many individuals feel unable to abstain totally from opiate drugs. As noted in chapter 1 in the discussion of conditioned withdrawal, detoxified opiate addicts report that the continued urges for opiates are associated with the subjective sensations of acute abstinence even though there may have been no actual exposure to opiates for weeks or months. This "narcotic hunger" has been hypothesized to be the driving force behind relapse to opiates.[5] Considered in this context, maintenance on methadone, an orally active, long-acting synthetic opiate, under medical supervision is a viable alternative to opiate addiction and all the social and medical consequences of such addiction (crime, AIDS, hepatitis, etc.). However, it is important to realize that the goal of methadone maintenance is rehabilitation, not abstinence, and there is strong evidence that methadone maintenance has restored thousands of hard-core addicts to responsible lives and has likely saved the lives of thousands more.[6]

The original research protocol for methadone maintenance was developed by Dole and Nyswander,[7] and subjects were selected based on severity of opiate addiction. The individuals had to have a 4 year history of heroin addiction with repeated attempts at detoxification followed by relapse. Subjects were also limited to the age group between 20 and 29 to eliminate younger addicts who might respond to other treatments and to eliminate older subjects because of the prevailing view that older subjects "grow out" of their addictions.

Treatment formed three distinct phases. In phase I, subjects were hospitalized for 6 weeks and started on small doses of oral methadone (10-20 mg/day), gradually increasing to a blocking level (80-120 mg/day). During phase II, the subjects were outpatients and returned to the clinic each weekday for medication and to leave a urine specimen. Methadone was dispensed orally in fruit juice. No formal psychotherapy was provided but the subjects received significant support and guidance from professional staff. Family adjustment and job placement became priorities. Once the subject made a successful transition from addict to patient and was productively engaged in normal outside activities, he entered phase III. Here, the maintenance dosage was continued with periodic review by a physician, and after careful review and evaluation, the well adjusted patients were allowed to visit the clinic once a week and to take home six bottles of methadone. Dole and Nyswander reported a program retention of 107 from 120 original patients, and 71% were employed in a steady job, in school or both.[8] Subsequently, research programs in New York City, Philadelphia and Washington, DC, all reported consistent success in stabilizing addicts on an ambulatory basis,[6] and in 1970, the Bureau of Narcotics and Dangerous Drugs, in a joint statement with the Food and Drug Administration, approved the use of methadone as an investigational drug for experimental maintenance programs.[9]

Modern guidelines for use of methadone suggest a wide range from 40-120 mg/day PO. Doses exceeding 60 mg/day are considered high-dose maintenance.[10] Low-dose maintenance has the advantage that, while side effects such as drowsiness are limited, craving produced by withdrawal is still blocked. High-dose maintenance not only has those characteristics but also provides a high enough dose to block any effects of heroin; e.g., heroin cannot override the receptor occupancy.

Subjects are first evaluated for objective signs of opiate withdrawal, and methadone is administered orally at a dose of 10 mg. The procedure is repeated every 2-4 hours and methadone administered as much as necessary for 24 hours, rarely more than 40 mg. At that point, the methadone dose is adjusted to a level at which the patient reports complete blockade of the effects of subsequently administered opiates, and random urine samples indicate that the use of opiates has stopped.

Patients on methadone maintenance are likely to come to the clinic daily and do not take drug home until evidence of significant rehabilitation is manifest. This type of compulsory clinic visit can facilitate subsequent counseling, psychotherapy, medical services and vocational programs that can help rehabilitation.

Methadone maintenance has the highest retention rate of any opiate treatment program.[10] It is the primary program for approximately 75,000 patients, and retention in the program at the 1 year point is 50-70%. Clear advantages include a reduction in illegal drug use and significant improvement in school and employment.

Problems in methadone maintenance are the continued use of illegal drugs and alcohol, diversion of methadone to illicit markets, and occasional overdose by those obtaining methadone illicitly.

OPPONENT PROCESS THEORY OF MOTIVATION AND OPIATE DEPENDENCE

Opiate dependence typically involves the development of tolerance and dependence, adaptive processes that are hypothesized to be the body's attempt to counter the acute effects of the drug. Such conceptualizations have been explored at all levels of opiate dependence research from the behavioral to the molecular.[11-14] The motivational hypothesis called "opponent process theory" has particular relevance to opiate dependence,[14,15] and recent studies have been designed to explore the neurobiological bases for opponent motivational processes using behavioral models to measure the motivational effects of drug withdrawal in animals.

Opponent process theory[15] postulates that affective states, pleasant or aversive, are automatically opposed by centrally mediated mechanisms that decrease the intensity of these affective states. Thus, positive reinforcers, such as acute administration of drugs, engage positive hedonic processes that are opposed by negative hedonic processes. The positive hedonic processes are hypothesized to be simple, stable and to follow administration of the drug closely in time. In contrast, negative hedonic processes are of longer latency, slow to build up strength, and slow to decay. Within this framework, the intense pleasure of the opiate "rush" or "high" is presumed to reflect a positive hedonic process, and the aversive withdrawal symptoms are presumed to reflect the opponent negative hedonic process.[13,14]

MOTIVATIONAL MEASURES OF OPIATE WITHDRAWAL

Withdrawal from chronic opiate administration is characterized by responses opposite to the acute initial actions of the drug (see above, especially chapter 1). Many of the overt *physical* signs associated with withdrawal from opiates can be easily quantified, while *motivational* measures require more than simple observation in many cases. Nevertheless, motivational measures are extremely sensitive measures of drug withdrawal. Animal models sensitive to the motivational effects of opiate withdrawal have included several different approaches, all of which measure some aspect of the negative affective state. Intracranial self-stimulation (ICSS) behavior has been used to assess changes in reward systems during the course of drug dependence. Acute administration of opiates increases the reward value of ICSS (for reviews see Kornetsky and Esposito[16] and Stellar and Rice[17]), and opiate withdrawal decreases the reward value of ICSS.[18-20] Operant schedules characterize the response-disruptive effects of drug withdrawal and provide a readily quantifiable measure of withdrawal (response rate).[21,22] Place aversion has been used to measure the aversive stimulus effects of withdrawal.[23,24] Rats exposed to a particular environment while undergoing withdrawal subsequently avoid that environment when presented with alternate environments. The elevated plus-maze provides a measure of anxiogenic-like responses associated with withdrawal. Animals are placed on an elevated cross-shaped platform that consists of closed and open arms. Precipitated withdrawal from morphine is characterized by increased time spent in the closed arms, similar to the response seen following stressor exposure or acute treatment with anxiogenic-like drugs.[25] Similar "anxiogenic-like" effects were observed using a defensive burying response during spontaneous opiate withdrawal.[26] Drug discrimination has also been used to characterize specific and nonspecific aspects of opiate withdrawal. Dependent animals can also be trained to discriminate low doses of naloxone from saline. During withdrawal, generalization to the naloxone cue suggests a withdrawal-like component to the withdrawal syndrome,[27,28] although this "withdrawal-like" cue is hard to separate from simply a non-morphine cue.[27] Each of these paradigms addresses a different theoretical construct associated with a given motivational aspect of withdrawal: some reflect more general malaise while others reflect more specific components of the opiate withdrawal syndrome.

NEUROBIOLOGICAL SUBSTRATES OF MOTIVATIONAL EFFECTS OF OPIATE WITHDRAWAL

As described in chapter 1 of this volume, opiate withdrawal in humans is characterized by a painful, flu-like state that includes many physical signs, but also consists of motivational ("purposive") signs of dysphoria and emotional discomfort. The classic *physical* signs of opiate withdrawal in rats are mediated by multiple sites of action, including the region of the locus coeruleus and its connections (see chapter 5). However, other regions in the basal forebrain such as the nucleus accumbens and amygdala have been implicated in the *motivational* effects of opiate withdrawal.[22,24,29]

Several studies have shown that withdrawal from opiate drugs decreases brain stimulation reward.[18-20] Spontaneous opiate withdrawal elevates brain stimulation reward thresholds.[19,20] Opiate withdrawal precipitated by naloxone is also characterized by elevations in reward thresholds.[18] Treatment of opiate-dependent rats with 1 mg/kg naloxone produced a significant elevation in thresholds[20] as measured by an auto-titration paradigm. More recently, opiate-dependent rats showed a profound sensitivity of morphine-dependent rats to naloxone in a discrete-trial, current-intensity threshold procedure[18] (Fig. 8.1). Consistent elevations in thresholds were seen in response to treatment with very low doses of naloxone (0.01 or 0.03 mg/kg SC). These were doses below which one observes major physical signs of opiate withdrawal, and treatment of nondependent rats with doses of naloxone as high as 1 mg/kg failed to significantly alter ICSS thresholds.

Using an operant schedule to measure the response-disruptive effects of precipitated opiate withdrawal produced some of the first insights into the substrates for the motivational effects of opiate withdrawal. Intracerebral microinjections of the hydrophilic opiate antagonist methylnaloxonium produced dose-dependent reductions in lever-pressing on a fixed ratio (FR)-15 operant schedule in opiate-dependent rats at doses that did not affect responding in nondependent rats. The most sensitive site for this opiate antagonist-induced disruption was the region of the nucleus accumbens,[22] a site also implicated in the acute reinforcing effects of opiates.[30] This disruption in operant responding occurred at doses of methylnaloxonium injected into the nucleus accumbens that failed to produce overt physical signs of withdrawal and thus was hypothesized to reflect the aversive affective properties of opiate withdrawal.

To directly test the hypothesis that the nucleus accumbens had a role in the aversive stimulus effects of opiate withdrawal, the conditioned place aversion test was used, combined with intra-

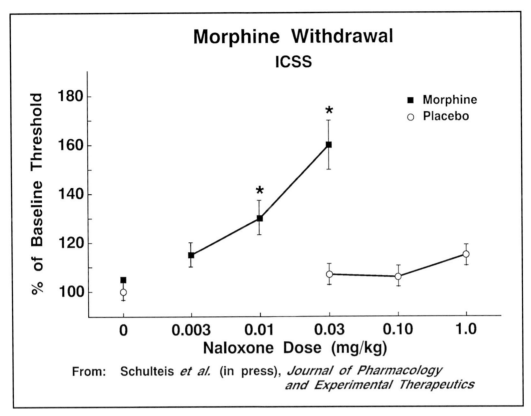

Fig. 8.1. Effects of precipitated opiate withdrawal on brain stimulation reward thresholds. Naloxone dose-dependently elevated brain stimulation reward thresholds in rats implanted with morphine pellets, but not in rats implanted with placebo pellets. The minimum dose of naloxone that elevated brain stimulation reward thresholds in the morphine group was 0.01 mg/kg [*p<0.05 vs. vehicle (V)]. Reproduced with permission from Schulteis G et al, J Pharmacol Exp Ther 1994; 271:1391-1398.

cerebral microinjections of methylnaloxonium in dependent rats.[24] Rats with bilateral cannulae aimed at the medial dorsal thalamus, periaqueductal gray, ventral tegmental area, amygdala or nucleus accumbens were made dependent on opiates and then subjected to place aversion training by pairing of a distinct environment (one of three arms of a box with distinct texture, markings and smell) with a single injection of methylnaloxonium. Injection of high methylnaloxonium doses (1,000-2,000 ng) produced a place aversion at all sites. However, injections of lower doses (250-500 ng) produced a significant effect only in the nucleus accumbens and amygdala, suggesting that these regions are critically involved in the aversive stimulus effects of opiate withdrawal (see Fig. 8.2).

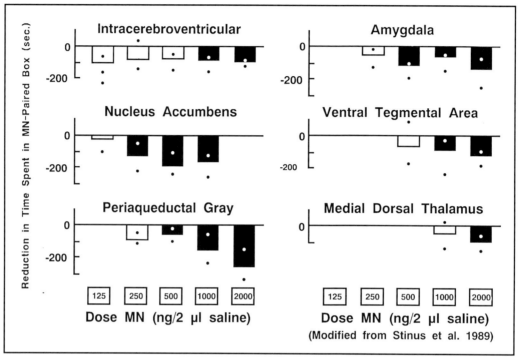

Fig. 8.2. The effect of intracerebral methylnaloxonium paired with a particular environment on the amount of time spent in that environment during an injection-free test session. Values represent the median difference between the postconditioning score and the preconditioning score. Dots denote the interquartile range of this distribution. Darkened bars represent doses at which the conditioning scores were significantly different from the preconditioning scores using the nonparametric Wilcoxon Matched Pairs Signed-Rank test. Level of significance was set at $p<0.02$ to control for multiple comparisons. Reproduced with permission from Stinus L et al, Neuroscience 1990; 37:767-773.

NEUROBIOLOGICAL MECHANISMS OF THE MOTIVATIONAL EFFECTS OF OPIATE WITHDRAWAL

Opiate tolerance and withdrawal involve not only physical signs but also changes in motivational state as described above. It has been hypothesized that there are two ways in which the brain reward system adapts to chronic drug insult: within-system and between-system neuroadaptations.[13] In a within-system adaptation, the primary cellular response responsible for the acute effects of the opiate would itself adapt to oppose and neutralize the drug's effects; persistence of the opposing effects after the drug disappears would produce the withdrawal response. In the between-system adaptation, different cellular and molecular systems from those involved in mediating the acute effects of the opiate, and triggered by the changes in the primary drug response neurons, would produce the tolerance and withdrawal after drug removal.

Within this framework, the neuropharmacological alterations in the postsynaptic elements of the opioid receptor, e.g., the intracellular messenger pathways (see chapter 3), could be considered a within-system adaptation.[31] Here, the same messenger system (adenylate cyclase, protein phosphorylation, etc.), presumably with an important, if not essential, role in the acute "hedonic"-like actions of opiates, may contribute to the motivational effects of cocaine withdrawal.

Possible neurotransmitter candidates in the nucleus accumbens involved in a between-systems adaptation include at this time acetylcholine, GABA, glutamate, corticotropin releasing factor, neuropeptide FF, CCK and dynorphin. The potential roles of neuropeptide FF, CCK and dynorphin were described in chapter 5. Acetylcholine release in the nucleus accumbens may be part of a between-systems adaptation in opiate withdrawal. Extracellular acetylcholine decreases after acute morphine injections. This effect shows tolerance with repeated administration, and during naloxone-precipitated opiate withdrawal, acetylcholine levels actually increase.[32]

Another possible example of a between-system adaptation to opiates may involve endogenous brain corticotropin releasing factor (CRF). CRF appears to have an important role in mediating behavioral responses to stressors and may be involved in the anxiogenic-like effects of ethanol withdrawal.[33,34] A CRF antagonist microinjected into the amygdala was able to block the place aversion produced by precipitated opiate withdrawal.[35]

Studies of cellular mechanisms of nociception have provided a model of the type of between-system adaptation that could also contribute to affective opponent processes.[36,37] Neurons in the rostral ventromedial medulla, "on-cells," that modulate nociception are depressed by morphine administration but show firing bursts just prior to an actual tail-flick reflex during analgesia testing. This on-cell activity correlates well with hyperalgesia. In contrast, "off-cells" in the rostral ventromedial medulla are activated by morphine but are silent or inactive during naloxone-precipitated hyperalgesia.[36] Opioid peptide and opiate excitation of off-cells is accompanied by an inhibition of the on-cell GABA inhibition,[37] suggesting that the hyperalgesic opponent response may involve an enhanced GABAergic transmission.

Another cellular example of neuroadaptation that is consistent with both within-system and between-system adaptations is the functional activity of the locus coeruleus and its inputs, some glutamatergic, during opiate withdrawal, as described in chapter 5 (see Akoaka and Aston-Jones,[38] Valentino and Aston-Jones[39]). At the molecular level, chronic opiate dependence is also associated with changes in second messenger systems not only in the locus coeruleus but also in the mesocorticolimbic dopamine system.[31] Identification of brain sites and neurochemical systems involved in the motivational effects of opiate withdrawal will allow better understanding of behavioral, cellular and molecular bases of opiate dependence.

SELF-MEDICATION CONTRIBUTION OF OPPONENT PROCESSES TO DEPENDENCE

Most views of drug dependence are focused upon the defining characteristic of compulsive, uncontrollable drug use; however, the basis for that compulsive use has been controversial. There are two major sources of reinforcement in drug dependence: positive reinforcement and negative reinforcement. One view is that the positive reinforcing effects of a drug are the major impetus for addiction. Clearly, positive reinforcing effects are critical for establishing self-administration behavior,[40,41] and alleviation of withdrawal symptoms is not likely to be a major motivating factor in the *initiation* of compulsive drug use. Neuroadaptation theories, such as opponent-process theory, postulate that the processes of affective habituation ("hedonic" tolerance) and withdrawal are the impetus for addiction. Clearly, this construct plays an important role in the *maintenance* of drug use after the development of dependence. Thus, while initial drug use may be motivated by the positive affective state produced by the drug, continued use leads to neuroadaptation to the presence of the drug and to the motivating properties of negative affective consequences of drug termination. Indeed, some have argued that the defining feature upon drug dependence is the establishment of a negative affective state.[42]

"The notion of dependence on a drug, object, role activity or any other stimulus-source requires the crucial feature of negative affect experienced in its absence. The degree of dependence can be equated with the amount of this negative affect, which may range from mild discomfort to extreme distress, or it may be equated with the amount or difficulty or effort required to do without the drug, object, etc." (Russell, pp. 184-185[42])

Defining drug addiction in this way leads directly to the concept of self-medication, and there are at least two ways that self-medication could form part of dependence. First, genetic or environmental factors could produce some neurobiological deficit that requires reversal. Alternatively, the chronic opiate-taking could produce a form of deficit state that requires self-medication to reverse. This type of deficit state can be hypothesized to exist at the molecular, cellular and system levels. One version of the molecular basis for such a need or deficit state was that chronic opiate administration produced an opioid peptide receptor down-regulation.[43] A more recent version would be that some intracellular messenger system on the postsynaptic side of this receptor would be responsible for this deficit state.[31] At the cellular level, as described above, one could hypothesize that some other neurotransmitter systems such as CRF or neuropeptide FF could contribute to the deficit state. At the system level, much evidence exists to suggest that the mesolimbic system, including dopamine and elements pre- and postsynaptic to the mesolimbic dopamine system, possibly incorporating elements of the amygdala or extended amygdala, may be the circuitry that supports not only the positive reinforcing effects of opiates but also the negative affective state associated with their withdrawal.[4]

The important question is how much of opiate dependence is driven by this deficit state. The success of methadone maintenance and the relative failure of opiate antagonist treatments speak to this issue (see above). However, it is clear that acute withdrawal and physical signs and symptoms do not drive dependence in detoxified addicts. There has to be some form of protracted abstinence syndrome that persists.

CONDITIONED REINFORCEMENT AND WITHDRAWAL

Drug dependence not only involves the acquisition and maintenence of drug-taking behavior, but also functions as a chronic relapsing disorder with reinstatement of drug-taking behavior after detoxification and abstinence. Both the positive and negative affective states can become associated with stimuli in the drug-taking environment through classical conditioning processes, motivating continued drug use and relapse after abstention upon re-exposure to these conditioned stimuli.

Conditioning to the positive affective states induced by drugs has been demonstrated in paradigms in which stimuli associated with drugs of abuse, including not only opiates but also psychomotor stimulants, nicotine, ethanol and barbiturates, can maintain responding in rats and monkeys when the stimulus is subsequently presented without the drug (for reviews see Markou et al[44] and Davis and Smith[45]). As with animals, there is evidence in humans that the positive reinforcing effects of heroin and cocaine, as measured by subjective reports of euphoria or "high," can become conditioned to environmental stimuli. Patients being treated for heroin addiction and allowed to self-administer either saline or heroin report that both saline and heroin injections were pleasurable, particularly in the patient's usual injection environment.[46] However, the conditioned feelings of "high" or euphoria were only reported after the actual injection, and many of these subjects reported feelings of withdrawal discomfort and dysphoria prior to injection, suggesting that conditioned withdrawal may also have motivational consequences.

Conditioned withdrawal has been repeatedly observed in opiate-dependent animals and humans. In the early classic studies by Wikler and colleagues,[47,48] rats made dependent by gradually increasing daily doses of morphine were exposed to a novel environment each night while experiencing morphine abstinence. After 6 weeks of such pairings, rats exposed to this same distinct environment showed *physical* withdrawal signs up to 155 days after the last morphine injection.

However, more importantly for the present discussion, *motivational* signs of withdrawal have been conditioned in animals. In rhesus monkeys made dependent and trained to lever-press for food on a FR-10 schedule, injection of the opiate-mixed agonist/antagonist nalorphine produced suppression of food-maintained responding and physical signs of withdrawal (reviewed in Goldberg[49]). After repeated pairings of a light or tone with the nalorphine injection, these conditioned stimuli alone could completely suppress responding. Similar results have also been obtained in morphine-dependent rats trained on a FR-15 schedule for food.[50] Here, responses to the conditioned stimulus persisted for one month after morphine termination by removal of subcutaneous morphine pellets.

Perhaps the most compelling evidence for the motivational properties of stimuli paired with opiate withdrawal is the observation that such stimuli actually come to influence drug-taking behavior. Monkeys allowed to intravenously self-administer morphine 24 hours per day were challenged once a day with repeated pairings of nalorphine and a light (reviewed in Goldberg[49]). Presentation of the light and injection of saline eventually resulted in a conditioned increase in responding for morphine, presumably to avert the onset of withdrawal. In a related study, lever-pressing terminated a green light that preceded infusion of an opiate antagonist and delayed antagonist injection for 60 seconds. Eventually, most of the responding occured during the period when the light cue was illuminated but before the antagonist was infused. These results are a powerful demonstration of the negative reinforcing properties of drug withdrawal.

As described in chapter 1, there is also significant clinical evidence of conditioned opiate withdrawal. Patients, even detoxified subjects, report symptoms like opiate abstinence when returning to environments similar to those associated with drug experiences.[51] Opiate addicts administered nalorphine on an irregular basis showed precipitated opiate abstinence,[52] and eventually placebo injections came to elicit similar withdrawal symptoms. Finally, such conditioned withdrawal can be elicited experimentally. Opiate addicts maintained on methadone[53] were given naloxone injections which were repeatedly paired with a tone and peppermint smell. Subsequent presentation of only the tone and odor elicited both subjective reports of discomfort and objective physical signs of withdrawal (see chapter 1 for details).

CONCLUSION: MOTIVATIONAL EFFECTS OF WITHDRAWAL

The present chapter has argued that, despite conceptual positions to the contrary,[40,41] the motivation for maintenance of compulsive opiate use involves negative reinforcement processes in addition to positive reinforcement processes. As discussed above, abstinence from opiates results in an aversive motivational state which can be quantified with a number of behavioral measures. These aversive motivational states are a dysregulator of motivational homeostasis and thus provide a mechanism for a negative reinforcement process where the organism is administering the drug to alleviate this aversive state.

Clearly, much remains to be explored about the neurobiology of the unconditioned negative motivational state(s) associated with opiates, particularly the conditioned negative motivational state(s). The study of the changes in the central nervous system associated with these homeostatic dysregulations may provide not only the key to opiate dependence, but also the key to the etiology of drug dependence in general and to the etiology of other psychopathologies associated with affective disorders.

REFERENCES

1. Koob GF. Animal models of drug addiction. In: Bloom FE, Kupfer DJ, eds. The Fourth Generation of Progress. New York: Raven Press, 1995:759-772.
2. American Psychiatric Association. Diagnostic and Statistical Manual of Mental Disorders, Fourth Edition. Washington, DC, American Psychiatric Association, 1995.
3. American Psychiatric Association. Diagnostic and Statistical Manual of Mental Disorders, Third Edition. Washington, DC, American Psychiatric Association 1980; 278-279.
4. Koob GF, Markou A, Weiss F et al. Opponent process and drug dependence: Neurobiological mechanisms. Semin Neurosci 1993; 5:351-358.
5. Dole VP. Narcotic addiction, physical dependence and relapse. N Engl J Med 1972; 286:988-992.
6. Lowinson JH. Methadone maintenance in perspective. In: Lowinson JH, Ruiz P, eds. Substance Abuse: Clinical Problems and Perspectives. Baltimore: Williams and Wilkins, 1981:344-354.
7. Dole VP, Nyswander M. A medical treatment for diacetylmorphine (heroin) addiction. J Am Med Assoc 1965; 193:646-650.

8. Dole VP, Nyswander M. Rehabilitation of heroin addicts after blockade with methadone. N Y State J Med 1966; 66:2011-2017.

9. Department of Health Education,and Welfare, and the Food and Drug Administration. New drugs: Conditions for investigational use of methadone for maintenance programs for narcotic addicts. Federal Register 1970; 35:9014-9015.

10. Gelenberg AJ, Bassuk EL, Schoonover SC. The Practitioner's Guide to Psychoactive Drugs. 3rd ed. New York: Plenum Publishing Corp., 1991.

11. Himmelsbach CK. Symposium: Can the euphoric, analgetic, and physical dependence effects of drugs be separated? IV. With reference to physical dependence. Fed Proc 1943; 2:201-203.

12. Collier HOJ. Cellular site of opiate dependence. Nature 1980; 283:625-630.

13. Koob GF, Bloom FE. Cellular and molecular mechanisms of drug dependence. Science 1988; 242:715-723.

14. Solomon RL. The opponent-process theory of acquired motivation: The affective dynamics of addiction. In: Maser JD, Seligman MEP, eds. Psychopathology: Experimental Models. San Francisco: W.H. Freeman and Co., 1977:124-145.

15. Solomon RL, Corbit JD. An opponent-process theory of motivation: 1. Temporal dynamics of affect. Psychol Rev 1974; 81:119-145.

16. Kornetsky C, Esposito RU. Euphorigenic drugs: Effects on reward pathways of the brain. Fed Proc 1979; 38:2473-2476.

17. Stellar JR, Rice MB. Pharmacological basis of intracranial self-stimulation reward. In: Liebman JM, Cooper SJ, eds. The Neuropharmacological Basis of Reward. Oxford: Clarendon Press, 1989:14-65.

18. Schulteis G, Markou A, Gold L et al. Relative sensitivity to naloxone of multiple indices of opiate withdrawal: A quantitative dose-response analysis. J Pharmacol Exp Ther 1994; 271:1391-1398.

19. Schaefer GJ, Michael RP. Morphine withdrawal produces differential effects on the rate of lever-pressing for brain self-stimulation in the hypothalmus and midbrain in rats. Pharmacol Biochem Behav 1983; 18:571-577.

20. Schaefer GJ, Michael RP. Changes in response rates and reinforcement thresholds for intracranial self-stimulation during morphine withdrawal. Pharmacol Biochem Behav 1986; 25:1263-1269.

21. Gellert VF, Sparber SB. A comparison of the effects of naloxone upon body weight loss and suppression of fixed-ratio operant behavior in morphine-dependent rats. J Pharmacol Exp Ther 1977; 201:44-54.

22. Koob GF, Wall TL, Bloom FE. Nucleus accumbens as a substrate for the aversive stimulus effects of opiate withdrawal. Psychopharmacology (Berlin) 1989; 98:530-534.

23. Hand TH, Koob GF, Stinus L et al. Aversive properties of opiate receptor blockade are centrally mediated and are potentiated by previous exposure to opiates. Brain Res 1988; 474:364-368.

24. Stinus L, Le Moal M, Koob GF. The nucleus accumbens and amygdala as possible substrates for the aversive stimulus effects of opiate withdrawal. Neuroscience 1990; 37:767-773.

25. Schulteis G, Markou A, Yackey M et al. Motivational consequences of naloxone-precipitated opiate withdrawal. NIDA Res Monogr 1995; 141(2):90. (Abstract)

26. Harris GC, Aston-Jones G. β-adrenergic antagonists attenuate withdrawal anxiety in cocaine- and morphine-dependent rats. Psychopharmacology 1993; 113:131-136.

27. France CP, Woods JH. Discriminative stimulus effects of naltrexone in morphine-treated rhesus monkeys. J Pharmacol Exp Ther 1989; 250:937-943.

28. Emmett-Oglesby MW, Mathis DA, Moon RTY et al. Animal models of drug withdrawal symptoms. Psychopharmacology 1990; 101:292-309.

29. Koob GF, Stinus L, Le Moal M et al. Opponent process theory of motivation: Neurobiological evidence from studies of opiate dependence. Neurosci Biobehav Rev 1989; 13:135-140.

30. Vaccarino FJ, Bloom FE, Koob GF. Blockade of nucleus accumbens opiate receptors attenuates intravenous heroin reward in the rat. Psychopharmacology 1985; 86:37-42.

31. Nestler EJ. Molecular mechanisms of drug addiction. J Neurosci 1992; 12:2439-2450.

32. Mark GP, Rada P, Pothos E et al. Is acetylcholine release in the nucleus accumbens part of a negative reinforcement process in drug withdrawal? Abstracts of the International Behavioral Neuroscience Society 1993; 2:20. (Abstract)

33. Baldwin HA, Rassnick S, Rivier J et al. CRF antagonist blocks alcohol withdrawal "anxiogenic" response. Psychopharmacology 1991; 103:227-232.

34. Rassnick S, Heinrichs SC, Britton KT et al. Microinjection of a corticotropin-releasing factor antagonist into the central nucleus of the amygdala reverses anxiogenic-like effects of ethanol withdrawal. Brain Res 1993; 605:25-32.

35. Heinrichs SC, Menzaghi F, Schulteis G et al. Suppression of corticotropin-releasing factor in the amygdala attenuates aversive consequences of morphine withdrawal. Behav Pharmacol 1995; 6:74-80.

36. Kim DH, Fields HL, Barbaro NM. Morphine analgesia and acute physical dependence: Rapid onset of two opposing dose-related processes. Brain Res 1990; 516:37-40.

37. Fields HL, Heinricher MM, Mason P. Neurotransmitters in nociceptive modulatory circuits. Annu Rev Neurosci 1991; 14:219-245.

38. Akaoka H, Aston-Jones G. Opiate withdrawal-induced hyperactivity of locus coeruleus neurons is substantially mediated by augmented excitatory acid input. J Neurosci 1991; 11:3830-3839.

39. Valentino RJ, Aston-Jones GS. Physiological and anatomical determinants of locus coeruleus discharge. In: Bloom FE, Kupfer DJ, eds. Psychopharmacology: The Fourth Generation of Progress. New York: Raven Press, Ltd., 1995:373-385.

40. Wise RA, Bozarth MA. A psychomotor stimulant theory of addiction. Psychol Rev 1987; 94:469-492.

41. Stewart J, De Wit H, Eikelboom R. Role of unconditioned and conditioned drug effects in the self-admininstration of opiates and stimulants. Psychol Rev 1984; 91:251-268.

42. Russell MAH. What is dependence? In: Edwards G, Russell MAH, Hawks D et al, eds. Drugs and Drug Dependence. Westmead, England: Saxon House/Lexington Books, 1976:182-187.

43. Dole VP. Implications of methadone maintenance for theories of narcotic addiction. JAMA 1988; 260:3025-3029.

44. Markou A, Weiss F, Gold LH et al. Animal models of drug craving. Psychopharmacology 1993; 112:163-182.

45. Davis WM, Smith SG. Conditioned reinforcement as a measure of the rewarding properties of drugs. In: Bozarth MA, ed. Methods of Assessing the Reinforcing Properties of Abused Drugs. New York: Springer-Verlag, 1987:199-210.

46. O'Brien CP, Greenstein R, Ternes J et al. Unreinforced self-injections: Effects of rituals and outcome in heroin addicts. In: Proceedings of the 41st Annual Meeting, Problems of Drug Dependence, L.S. Harris (ed). NIDA Res Monogr 1979; 27:275-281.

47. Wikler A, Pescor FT. Classical conditioning of a morphine abstinence phenomenon, reinforcement of opioid-drinking behavior and "relapse" in morphine addicted rats. Psychopharmacologia 1967; 10:255-284.

48. Wikler A. Dynamics of drug dependence: Implications of a conditioning theory of research and treatment. Arch Gen Psychiatry 1973; 28:611-616.

49. Goldberg SR. Stimuli associated with drug injections as events that control behavior. Pharmacol Rev 1976; 27:325-340.

50. Baldwin HA, Koob GF. Rapid induction of conditioned opiate withdrawal. Neuropsychopharmacology 1993; 8:15-21.

51. O'Brien CP. Experimental analysis of conditioning factors in human narcotic addiction. Pharmacol Rev 1976; 27:533-543.

52. Wikler A, Fraser HF, Isbell M. N-allynormorphine: Effects of single doses and precipitation of acute "abstinence syndromes" during addiction to morphine, methadone or heroin in man (post-addicts). J Pharmacol Exp Ther 1953; 109:8-20.
53. O'Brien CP, Jesta J, O'Brien TJ et al. Conditioned narcotic withdrawal in humans. Science 1977; 195:1000-1002.

INDEX

Page numbers in italics denote figures (f) or tables (t).

DATE DUE

NOV 1 7 1998 MAY 1 7 2000	
DEC 0 2 1998	
APR 1 2 1999	
MAY 2 7 1999	
APR 1 4 2010	
MAY 0 4 2010	